For information, contact:

christophersalah@yahoo.com

Library of Congress Catalog-in-Publication Data

Salah, Christopher.
One less excuse: concise, up-to-date, scientifically proven & researched information to take back your health /
Christopher Salah.
Includes index.
TXu 1-872-933

ISBN: 978-1-4675-9930-6 (sc)
ISBN: 978-1-4675-9931-3 (e)

Cover Design & Layout: Nikki Orzel

The contents and information in this book are not substitutes for competent and personal medical care. Any diet or lifestyle changes implemented by a reader of this book are adopted at the sole discretion and risk of that individual reader. Modifications to diet and lifestyle should be monitored by your doctor. All the information in this book has been gained through scientific research and an expert knowledge of the physiology of the human body. If your doctor is not open to the information here it might be time to find a physician who is more open and interested in your health.

Lovingly dedicated to:

My mother, father and entire family for their unwavering support

Nikki, for breathing life into my book and making it a reality

Porter, for going above and beyond

Andrea, for the countless times she patiently read and re-read the proofs along with her inspirational insight

About the Author

I come from a very conservative family. Although I know my parents would have supported me in any career path, it felt that my main choices were doctor, lawyer or "do what Dad does." Dad was in the hotel business, which was not for me. My sister was a lawyer, and she made it clear that field wasn't for me either. So doctor it was. However, I'm not sure how I knew it at the time, but I knew for sure that having a nurse take your vitals and spending one to two minutes with the doctor before he or she handed you pills to take…was not medicine. I wanted to help people be healthy and stay healthy; full of energy and life. It was actually my sister who handed me the brochure for the school in Los Angeles that offered a degree in Chinese medicine. I was fifteen years old when this happened.

After high school I quickly finished my two-year Associate's and started a two-thousand-hour program to obtain a Master's of Science in Oriental Medicine. The medicine was amazing. Although I am known as an acupuncturist, this is actually a poor title for people with my degree. We spend more hours of study learning hundreds upon hundreds of herbs and the combination of these herbs to treat illness. Just like doctors use pharmaceuticals, we use herbs — except we aim to treat the root of the condition and not just mask the symptoms of a disease. We learned all types of different techniques to encourage the body to heal itself. Our training also focused on meditation, exercise programs, nutrition, and everything we needed to help people prevent disease and heal the body.

After I finished my Master's, I spent years working alongside orthopedic surgeons as part of a team doing post-op rehabilitation. It was amazing to see that the people who elected to have me as part of their team healed twice as fast and used half their medications. It was here that I started to notice the impact that stress has on the body. It was quite obvious that my patients who felt more stress — because of the circumstances involving surgery — did not heal as fast.

A couple of years later I enrolled in a clinical doctorate program while maintaining a private practice and continuing to work with the surgeons. As part of my doctorate I started to teach Chinese medicine, discovering that teaching was a passion of mine. I have been teaching in one form or another ever since. During my doctorate years, I spent time in hospitals and community clinics, treating everyone from the homeless person you see every day to the people who have never worked a day in their lives. From the very poor to the very rich; tens of thousands of people crossed my path and every day I helped them as best I could.

Through so much interaction with my patients, their bodies, and their health; with miracle successes and miserable failures, I started to see patterns in who the healthy people were and who the ill were. I saw patterns in who healed faster, who responded better to treatment, and who did not.

It became glaringly obvious that there are two major aspects of life that influence our health strongly; stress and diet. These were the core principles ingrained in the philosophy of Chinese medicine but, over the years, I had started to lose my way and not completely address these factors wholeheartedly. I had become too focused on trying to fix people instead of giving my patients the knowledge to fix themselves.

Knowing that eating well is the foundation for our health, I wanted to be able to answer any and all of my patients' questions. I wanted to be able to guide them in the right direction. To accomplish this, I went to the bookstore and bought about a dozen of the best-selling diet and nutrition books out there: books by Dr. Mehmet C. Oz, Dr. Dean Ornish, Dr. Andrew Weil, John Robinson, Dr. Jessica K. Black, T. Colin Campbell, Ph.D., and Thomas M. Campbell II to name a few. What was astonishing was that the information and research contained in these books was the same — 90% of the time, all these doctors agreed! This is shocking in the medical world.

Then a change of life happened. I am an adventurous person at heart. Although I absolutely love what I do — being able to help people live happier, healthier lives — I was bored with *my* life.

One day at school between the classes I was teaching, I saw a poster that read, “How would you like to see the world and do what you love?” It was from a company that placed acupuncturists on cruise ships. I decided to call, and six months later I was flying to Sydney, Australia, to join my first ship's crew.

Over the next year, this would become the main motivator to write and publish the information in this book.

Part of my job on the ships was to lecture and educate the guests about alternative medicine and health in general. Every single week for nine months I did a lecture on diet and nutrition based on the most current scientific research available. Thousands of people took a seat to listen, and every single week I startled people with this information. Week after week, month after month, I got surprised looks and the same questions over and over.

Now, after almost three years of lecturing and helping Australian, British, and American cruise passengers, I know it wasn't just my American patients at home who needed help. Almost everyone I met who suffered from any form of illness had no clue how to take care of their bodies and correct the imbalances that made them suffer. Many simply took pills that their doctors gave them to keep them alive just a little bit longer.

This book is dedicated to dispelling the collective ignorance to which we (including my former self) are slaves. I have done this by compiling thousands upon thousands of pages of health science, translating it into a language everyone can understand, and writing a short and simple book that addresses the core issues in our lives. I hope everyone who reads this will find something in it that benefits his or her life; something to make life easier, more comfortable, and more enjoyable.

In my mind there is nothing worse than living sick, in pain, and worrying about or managing a disease. After a decade of service to others, I know firsthand that if we know the right information and if we use it, we can regain our health. I will start this book exactly how I will end it.

Never give up!

About This Book

Having lectured on health topics on three continents I've been asked hundreds of times after my seminars, “Have you written a book?” My answer was always the same, “No” because everything I present has already been written. All the facts are out there. The studies, the research, have all been done. Information on health and diet has been published over and over. There are our famous doctors on TV sharing the same information that I present in my lectures. There are documentaries and films; CDs and DVDs. Yet week after week and month after month, the majority of people and patients I speak to, including my own family, are still very, very confused as to what goes into good health. What does it include? Where do we start?

My last little nudge to "write about something already written" came when I was doing house calls. Time after time, I would walk in to see a patient and out of the corner of my eye see the book I'd recommend sitting on the shelf collecting dust. When I go to my family's and friends' houses, I'd see the same books because I either recommended them, they saw them on TV, or someone else said they loved them. But there the books sat with their first 20 pages creased, no more, placed forever in the corner. More times than not, when I gave a book recommendation, my patients would tell me they already had that one. Did you read it? The answer, usually: no.

The reason for this is fairly simple. Many of us, including myself, are lazy when it comes to our health and most good books by famous and distinguished doctors are too long.

They are technical, written in scientific terms, and they can be dense and confusing. This is especially true if you know nothing about the human body and how it functions.

The following is both the disclaimer for this book, a description of exactly what this book offers, and how it can help you and your loved ones enjoy improved health and better lives.

This book is not intended to diagnose, treat, prevent, or cure any illness or disease and does not replace competent medical care by a qualified practitioner. Funny enough, the information in this book has been scientifically proven to treat, cure, and quite specifically prevent disease in the human body. However, it is important that any changes to diet or lifestyle be monitored by your physician especially if you are taking medications for life-threatening illnesses. Unfortunately many physicians are not trained or educated in the topics presented in this book, and like many of us have been corrupted to think only one way about diet and lifestyle. If your current doctor is not open to the information presented here then it is time to consider finding one who is more open, up-to-date, and supportive of what you're trying to do as someone courageously embracing health and happiness.

What's in this book? This book is a compilation of many famous doctors' work, cutting-edge scientific researchers' observations, the writings of best-selling authors on health and diet, along with basic human physiology (how the body works) — all tied together into a simple, easy-to-understand program to move you forward into general well-being and health. Everything in this book is supported by scientific research (almost all of it from human trials). There is a "notes" section in the back that says where a particular quote was found. And Appendix E is a further-reading section with the most cutting-edge and informational books.

Many will feel that what is presented here is too “out there” and fantastic because for so many years we've been told otherwise by our parents, doctors and people we trust. There will be a lot in this book that goes against what we've always known and believed. I urge you to be open and know that everything written here has been proven to be true through research; research done on individuals, on societies, and even on entire populations.

Chapter 1

Let's Look At Some Facts

Americans spend more money per person on health care then any other country in the world, yet our nation is ranked 37th in health-care performance, 27th in life expectancy, and our health is getting worse and worse. Heart disease is the number one killer and will claim the lives of one out of three Americans. After heart disease, the second leading cause of death is cancer. Just five years ago when educating my patients, I used to say that one out of three of us will get cancer; now, that statistic is one in two. Obesity has doubled in the United States in the last 30 years: one-third of Americans are obese and more than 60 percent are overweight. Diabetes, one of the Top 10 killers, has increased 70 percent in people in their 30s from 1990 to 1998 resulting in 25.8 million Americans suffering with diabetes by 2010! I see too many of my patients in their 60s and 70s who are completely overwhelmed with sickness and disease. Take a second to read this paragraph again and imagine what we are doing to ourselves — and what our children, our society looks like if we get so sick so much earlier in our lives.

Excuse Not To Change #1

I will spare you the numbers but I could most likely be able to fill another book with how bad our health is and how, year by year, we get worse. Most of us will know a lot of this already so it shouldn't be a surprise. The problem is that many of us don't want to change and adopt a healthy lifestyle because we have too much faith in the current medical system.

When I speak on health and diet, one of the biggest arguments I get from people who don't want to change is this: "It's only because of modern medicine that we are living longer and longer." This is true to some extent. The current medical system is largely pharmaceutical-based. It is these drugs that are keeping us alive amid the diseases with which we suffer.

Facts: After heart disease and cancer one of the biggest threats to our health is medical care. Adverse side effects from drugs, hospital-borne infections, unnecessary surgeries and medical errors combine to be the third leading cause of premature death in our country!

Our system is broken. We have given away our right to be healthy and entrusted it to the drug companies that are barely keeping us alive. Drug companies are in business for one reason; to make money, hit targets and keep their investors happy. Do you think they really care about your health? No! Therefore, if drug companies have no interest in your health and we get our drugs from our doctors, then who is really watching over your health, your body and your life?

I would really like to think that this information will change the lives of millions of people. In reality though, it is my hope that at the very least everyone who reads this understands that we are sheep to the pharmaceutical companies and that there are many aspects to our lives that we can change on our own to be healthy.

With all that said, are we really living longer? One of the first things that my patients hand me is a list of their medications. In fact, I keep some of these at home on my wall for my own motivation. My long-lived patients hobble in with arthritis; they have trouble walking because of theirs knees; they can't open jars or work in the yard because of their hands; they have back pain, urinary problems that keep them up at night, digestive issues, and vision problems, let alone what starts to happen to the mind. Compare this to my proactive patients and the many people I have met along the way who take care of themselves and who are still very much alive and active. Who's really living longer?

I'll never forget the Christmas Eve that I was sitting on the couch with my dad and out of the blue he said he never thought things would end up like this. Both of my parents on separate occasions have voiced the fact that they are just waiting to die. That they never thought they would live this long. It's terrible to watch my Mom struggle to climb the single flight of stairs in our old house, out of breath and in pain. Both my parents and my patients take handfuls of pills in the morning, some at lunch to protect them from the toxic effects of the ones in the morning, and then another handful at night because the other medications cause insomnia, depression, anxiety, and tummy troubles. Even if this does not sound like you yet, statistics show that unless we start accepting responsibility for our health, most of us will end up like this. All you have to do is look around you.

If you are still not convinced and carry a torch for modern medicine, then think about this — especially if you have children. The following quotation is from Eric M. Bost, Undersecretary for Food, Nutrition, and Consumer Services for the USDA before the House Committee on Government Reform, in 2004.

> *Recent trends among children are alarming: In the past 20 years, the percentage of children who are overweight has doubled and the percentage of adolescents who are overweight has more than tripled. If we do not stem this tide, many children in this generation of children will not outlive their parents.*

This is quitc possibly the first time in our nation's history that our life span may actually have started to get shorter, making the argument that modern medicine has increased our life expectancy null and void.

What modern medicine has done so well is keep us living with diseases that we inflict on ourselves. Would you hand your child a cigarette? I'll never forget a particular seminar in which there was a screaming 2-year-old in the back. Mom, who was obese, quickly produced a bag of potato chips, opened them (because the 2-year-old would not have been able to do this on his own) and gave them to the toddler. There is no difference in this story than handing your child a cigarette. Both are addictive and both cause disease.

Change is hard. I'm no saint, either, and I will share some of my personal stories throughout. Even if you are unable to make the changes yourself you should know that if you're a parent, you're deciding the fate of your children's health by what you feed them and how they're educated at home. If you don't take action, the food and drug companies will do it, and that is the source of the confusion for all of us.

Keep reading and take back your health and the health of your children and your future. It's never too late.

Excuse Not To Change #2

"My parents both had heart disease, my grandfather had diabetes, and both my grandmother and mom had breast cancer. So what's the point? I am going to die of these anyway so I might as well enjoy myself."

The fact is that genetics only account for about 5 percent of disease transmission.

Now, this needs to be explained because it does not mean that you will not get these genes. Genes are similar to light switches. Millions of times a day these little switches are turned on and turned off in different sequences to do different things. We get sick when at a certain point in time a certain gene gets "stuck" either on or off. Medical science has shown that only 5 percent of us will get genes for diseases that get stuck all by themselves. The rest of us decide what they do every minute of our lives.

Everything you eat, every time you exercise or don't, drink water or not, smoke or take drugs — all of this decides what these genes are doing. If we do something that triggers these genes for long enough at some point, they will get stuck and we get sick. For example, if your parents had early arthritis, then you most likely have the genes for it too, but what you do with your life decides whether they turn on. The same goes for heart disease, hypertension, diabetes, cancer, and so on. When you eat your veggies and exercise, the chances of turning on the cancer gene decreases. When you smoke and eat lots of meat, the chances of turning on the cancer gene increases. This is how it works. Genes are absolutely no excuse not to take care of yourself.

Excuse Not To Change #3

One word: ignorance. Why is everyone so confused? Because keeping you ignorant and confused is big money. Companies spend billions of dollars advertising so you'll buy their food. It should be obvious too that they don't care about your health. If they did, then you wouldn't see companies advertising food that kills you, but we do see those commercials every minute of every day. A great example is milk. We see milk ads at least every half-hour on TV, let alone on billboards and in magazines. That's a lot of money. Who cares, though? — milk is healthy and good for you… right? Ironically, the only reason you know milk is healthy is because of the millions of dollars spent each year on advertising telling you it is.

Milk is not all it's cracked up to be, and there is a whole discussion on dairy later in the book. But for now, let's stay with what we know. We know that almonds are healthy and if you look at a package of almonds you will see a health claim from the American Heart Association that says scientific evidence suggests that almonds in your diet can help prevent heart disease. We know that fiber is essential for our bodies and is good for us. That's why on a box of Cheerios® and other cereals, you will see a health claim saying that scientific evidence suggests a diet high in fiber helps prevent heart disease. Go get the milk carton from your fridge and look at it. Do you see any health claims? No, because not only is there no science to show that milk is healthy for any part of your body, what we will see later is that it's actually detrimental to your health.

Many people already know this and are starting to switch over to alternatives like soy, almond and rice milk. Now what are we seeing on TV? Advertisements against these alternatives that actually make you feel stupid for switching. This is exactly what they're intended to do. This phenomenon happens in every arena from the meat industry to the grain industry and in between, which is why we stay confused.

One Less Excuse is dedicated to dispelling these myths and presenting only information that has scientific evidence. While you read this, try to set aside the things you have heard or believe to know. Keep an open mind, and this information will absolutely make sense to you. Although there is new scientific research, sadly enough most of the statements and facts in this book have been around and publicized for at least 50 years. Whether you start to make changes for a healthy and vibrant life, at least next time you wake up you will know the truth.

Chapter 2

The Biggest Threats to Our Health

I'm sorry, I'm sorry, I'm sorry. Before we get into this let me just say: I have won blue ribbons in cooking competitions for my baby back pork ribs. Nothing makes my mouth water more than a bacon cheese burger and I'll easily take down a whole Meat Lover's® pizza by myself. The fact is that there is undeniable evidence backed by hundreds if not thousands of scientific studies, both on animals and humans, both in the lab and throughout entire religions and cultures the world round that proves…

Animal products are the biggest detriment to our health as human beings. Meat and meat products promote heart disease, cancer, heart attacks, high blood pressure, high cholesterol, kidney disease, and osteoporosis.

Starting simple, what is meat? Advertising has kept us ignorant in thinking that red meat, mainly cow, is "meat." Here's my dad's story.

After he had a triple bypass and a heart-valve replacement, I went to stay with him and help with his recovery. The first thing we talked about was eliminating as much meat from his diet as possible. He looked at me and said, "Baby (I'll never outgrow that) your mom and I don't eat that much meat. For breakfast, we might have some cereal. Lunch will be a wrap with just a little turkey or ham and cheese. For dinner, Mom and I have either chicken or fish." Look again at the quote above. It says "meat and meat products." This is what most of us don't understand. It's the protein from animal products that's creating disease.

The milk on my dad's cereal is considered a meat product because it contains animal protein. The ham and turkey both had eyes at some point in life and, although more lean, are still meat. For that matter, so is the cheese in the wrap. Meat on meat. Then there is the fish. Yes, it's lean. Yes, it's healthier cholesterol-wise than red meat, but fish is still an animal with a face and family and what you are eating is the muscle tissue of that animal. Therefore it is meat. I have only been in one argument in which I lost my cool with a patient and that was a half-hour discussion about fish being considered meat. Last, but not least: eggs. Why they are considered dairy, I have no idea. If that egg was fertilized and you gave it back to its mother it will turn into a chicken, which is an animal, making it meat. So you see that between the red meat we indulge in, chicken, turkey, fish, milk, cheese, butter, and eggs, most of us eat animal products all day long.

Before I personally embraced this information, I had these arguments with vegetarians.

Humans have canines and incisors. Only animals that eat meat have these types of teeth. We also have the flatter molars for vegetation indicating the fact that we are supposed to be omnivores; eating both flesh and vegetation. We have one stomach and a fairly short digestive tract, again pointing to being able to eat both types of food. Pure meat-eating animals have even shorter digestive tracts. We have enzymes that rapidly and effectively digest animal products, and virtually no enzymes to digest plant matter. With all this said, then why would there be an unbelievable amount of evidence absolutely concluding that animal products create disease?

Plain and simple: we eat too much animal and not enough vegetable.

We do not eat the balance of meat and vegetables that our bodies were designed for. In the past we had to hunt for it. In many cultures, it is only eaten on special occasions. It is a relatively new phenomenon whereby we can stop at a fast-food joint on the way to work and grab sausages and eggs. Grab a sandwich or wrap for lunch, and then go to the store and buy some type of meat for dinner. Our bodies are not meant for such a high consumption of animal products.

How much meat should we be eating for optimum health? Five percent of your total daily caloric intake. For a 2,000-calories-a-day diet this is about 25 grams of protein (3 to 4 ounces of meat) – it would fit into a cupped hand. The Germans have always been renowned for their athletes. Over 60 years ago, German scientists found that protein intake for peak athletic performance and recovery was 60 to 80 grams. Our government has always been a little slow to respond to changing trends, but if you go to the USDA web site and look at the new food guidelines, you'll see that protein intake has been lowered to 64 grams per day for a person weighing 175 pounds. In addition, the World Health Organization (WHO) agrees that protein intake should account for between 10 and 15 percent (50 to 75 grams or about 7 ounces) of total caloric intake. This is a small serving of meat or animal product for only one meal per day.

Where did the lower number, the 5 percent, come from? It came from two places.

Research shows the lowest incidence of premature death from most major diseases when animal protein is at or below 5 percent. The second is a little more fascinating than science — it came from human beings. Mothers' milk, the same milk that is supposed to nourish a newborn baby during its most delicate time of incredible growth and change, consists of only 5 percent protein. This could not be a more poignant message from nature. Hopefully by now you can see that in our modern society, we eat way, way too much meat and animal products. But is it really that bad for us?

Facts: Vegetarians have lower rates of heart disease, 50 percent less.

Vegetarians have lower rates of cancer, obesity, hypertension, diabetes, kidney and colon disease.

Yet the meat and dairy companies push and push, through billion-dollar ad campaigns, the message that we cannot survive, let alone be healthy, without their products.

Facts: Cardiovascular disease, the No. 1 killer, is virtually nonexistent in populations that don't consume meat.

For awhile, scientists thought there might be a genetic component to these populations, but the Seventh-Day Adventists prove otherwise. This is a religion, not a race, which practices vegetarianism. Additionally, we see populations which immigrate to the U.S., adopt our diet and then start having the same rates of heart disease we do. From the Framingham Heart Study, one of the longest-running health studies ever conducted on humans, we know that people who have a cholesterol value of 150 or lower do not have to worry about heart attacks.

Facts: The average American cholesterol is 210

The average vegetarian cholesterol is 161

The average vegan cholesterol is 133

"*Nothing will benefit human health and increase chances for survival of life on Earth as much as the evolution to a vegetarian diet*"

–Albert Einstein

Facts: The average IQ of vegetarian children is higher by almost 20 points than their meat-eating counterparts.

The facts are simple, straightforward, and astonishing: people who eat a more animal-based diet suffer from more disease and illness. People who have a more plant-based diet have less.

But why?

There are several reasons why eating so much animal product causes disease. If more protein is eaten than what our body can use, it is broken down into toxic chemicals by our liver. I'm always amazed at the number of people I see in my office who have high liver enzymes and/or a fatty liver but don't drink or smoke. It's because this excessive amount of animal protein damages the liver. These chemicals are then excreted by the kidneys, which also suffer. Studies show increased rates of kidney disease in people who consume a high-protein diet. In fact, liver and kidney damage are "side effects" of the now-debunked Atkins diet.

Animal protein stimulates the liver to produce excessive amounts of cholesterol. This is a little-known biological fact I learned in my first year of physiology in college. This is embarrassing and a shame for many of our doctors out there. Sixteen percent of Americans – more than 30 million — have high cholesterol. When you get that blood test back that says you have high cholesterol, if you have a good doctor, he or she will tell you to try diet and exercise before they put you on drugs, drugs you'll have to take for the rest of your life. Your doctor's advice is to lower cholesterol in your diet typically by eating less red meat, more lean meats such as fish and avoiding creams, butters, and products high in cholesterol and saturated fat.

Six months later, you go back to your doctor and get checked again but your cholesterol is still high. Now you have to start taking the drugs which have toxic side effects. What most doctors fail to tell you is that cholesterol is so important to your body that your liver can make every single little bit of cholesterol *even if you do not eat any in your diet*.

HEART DISEASE PUZZLE PIECE #1 Eating animal-based products (animal protein) triggers the liver to make excessive amounts of cholesterol. So even eating a chicken breast or switching to non-fat milk can elevate your cholesterol levels. This is how eating too much protein (over 5 ounces a day) contributes to high cholesterol, stroke, heart disease, and heart attack.

Milk and Milk Products

Although milk is included in the above information on meat and meat products, it is such a silent threat that it requires it own discussion. It's "silent" because most of us believe that it's healthy and necessary for our bodies. Again, let me start out by saying that cheese and ice cream are two of my favorite things on this planet. Unfortunately the science is there and you cannot ignore the facts.

Facts: No other animal on our planet consumes milk after infancy, let alone cross-species milk. You do not see pigs sucking on cows, so why should we?

Milk contains a protein called casein that has been proven to be carcinogenic (cancer promoting).

Scientific studies show that milk and milk products increase the risk of suffering from heart disease, diabetes, prostate and ovarian cancers, and obesity.

Speaking of obesity, did you know that a baby cow can gain over 350lbs in one year just from drinking its mother's milk? We also know that milk is a substance that produces mucus in the body. More than 50 percent of most populations are intolerant to milk. In other people, even if they can digest it, we know that it triggers an immune response. If a child suffers from allergies and/or asthma, the first thing that should be done is to have that child stop consuming dairy products. Yet this is rarely done.

Even without the fat, as in low-fat or non-fat milk, the protein casein is still there. On top of that, when you take out the fat you also take out all the nutrients, essentially creating white protein water. Go to your fridge and look at the ingredients. You will see that the vitamin A and D have been added because it is the fat in the milk that has these vitamins.

The last problem is that almost all the nutrients and enzymes that could be beneficial for you have been destroyed by homogenization and pasteurization. Here's a fun science experiment. Take a glass of whole raw milk just like nature intended and set it out on the counter next to the white stuff you get from the store. Cover with a paper towel. After a couple of days you will notice that the real milk has started to separate into two things, two new, perfectly edible foods called curds and whey. The stuff from the store will not do this; it will rot and become unsafe to drink.

When I lecture on this topic hands start to go up as soon as I finish my last sentence. Nothing generates such a response from the audience than when I speak about milk. When the hands go up, the questions are always the same. "If we're going to believe you, then where are we going to get our calcium?" My response is always quick and with a smile. "Where do the cows get their calcium?"

Many, many vegetables on our planet provide high amounts of calcium. All dark green leafy vegetables have calcium and ones like kale, Brussels sprouts and broccoli have more bio-available calcium than milk. Many nuts and seeds also have calcium, notably almonds. Not only have you been kept in the dark about milk, but you've been blatantly lied to. There is no scientific evidence that milk increases bone density and prevents osteoporosis. In fact, it's quite the opposite. For women sometime after the age of 40, there will be a day when a doctor does a bone density test. If your test comes back with poor bone density, you're told to consume more dairy before you're put on drugs. A year later you return for another test and not only are the results not better, they're worse. Here's why.

Milk is high in animal protein. Animal protein, including milk, creates an acidic environment inside the body. The body does not like to be acidic so it buffers it with calcium carbonate and excretes the waste through the urine. By drinking milk you are actually losing more calcium than you're getting, which is why we see high rates of osteoporosis in a country that consumes so much dairy. Osteoporosis and kidney disease, which are high in the U.S., are signs of excess protein intake, which includes dairy.

Facts: In a very large study done on nurses, the evidence shows that there was a higher rate of bone fractures within the group that drank more milk per week.

Another, separate study, showed that in the elderly, the ones who consumed the most milk per week actually had double the risk for hip fractures.

Daily exercise is far more important for strong bones, especially the weight bearing type that strengthens muscles.

No more excuses. Basic human physiology, hundreds of scientific studies, and thousands upon thousands of research hours have absolutely proven that the standard American diet that is high in animal products causes disease. It causes us to suffer unnecessarily and costs billions of dollars in health care. That's money that we could use for other more important needs in our society. But, can you really regain your health, even if you already suffer from these diseases? Is it too late for change?

Chapter 3

Understanding Health

Millions of Americans are clueless when it comes to their bodies and their health. Because of this, our bodies slowly start to change and we start to get sick. Blood pressure starts to go up, blood sugar is unbalanced, arteries start to clog, cancers start to form; we get tired, can't sleep, get depressed, and live in pain. A trip to the doctor and now we have to take drugs that do not fix us. We have to take drugs that simply alter our chemistry and mask these symptoms; symptoms of a deeper underlying problem. Then, most of us have to take these drugs for the rest of our lives.

The worst part about this is that there exists an even deeper secret: our collective ignorance, which includes many of our doctors, goes beyond putting too much faith in pharmaceutical drugs. It's about not taking responsibility for our own health. The sad truth is that we are sold on modern medicine and have given up our right to choose to be healthy and disease free!

Is this an overstatement? If I told you that some cancers can be stopped by changing your diet and most can be prevented even if it runs in the family; would you believe me? If I told you that type 2 diabetes can be reversed even if you're taking medications, would you believe me? How about if I told you that heart disease can be stopped? — not only stopped but also reversed? Or if I told you the plaque clogging your arteries can go away and that you can do all this yourself? Would you believe me?

Ninety percent of the people who attend my seminars do not believe it could be this simple. It's very much the same in my private practice. Too many of us have given up our power of free thought to big corporations that tell us what we should eat. We have given up our free thought to our doctors who tell us what drugs to take. Every year it's something new, something different, some different advice that the next year turns out was wrong. So when the question is asked – "Is it too late to change?" — let's start with what should worry us most. The No. 1 disease of which Americans die prematurely…

Heart Disease

Over 1 million Americans will undergo a coronary bypass or angioplasty for clogged arteries every year. This costs us and our health care system over $15 billion annually. This money could go to our failing school system, public works, or any number of more important avenues to improve our lives. The worst part about this is that almost half of us will once again have clogged arteries within six months after the procedures if we continue to eat a meat based diet, don't exercise, and don't manage our stress.

But numbers are just numbers until it hits home. A couple of years back I got a call from my sister telling me that my dad just got back from an ordinary routine physical and that his heart was so bad that they scheduled him for surgery the next day! After a triple bypass and a heart-valve replacement he was still alive, and a couple of days later he was home. I went to see him a week later to see if I could help.

Two things I'll never forget. He was weak and couldn't change himself. Helping him one night into his pajamas I can still see the eight inch incision where they split his ribcage in half to get to his heart. I cannot imagine having to make a decision in which my only option is being split in half and opened up. The next memory I have: helping him into bed every night and tucking him in. I do not posses the literary skill to describe the feeling of how wrong it felt in my heart to tuck my dad into bed, especially knowing that this could have been avoided.

One of the best-known doctors in this field is Dr. Dean Ornish. Through comprehensive human clinical trials, Dr. Ornish has proven beyond a doubt that by changing diet and lifestyle, we can stop and even reverse heart disease. His research indicates that people with heart disease not only get significant health benefits but longer-lasting results with these changes as well. Most importantly, he has shown that following his program for at least a year, 80 percent of patients, even severe cases, can avoid surgery altogether! Please re-read this paragraph and understand that the No. 1 cause of premature death can be stopped and corrected without surgery or drugs.

The unfortunate part of this is that although Dr. Ornish is probably the most notable, other doctors have proven the same thing years ago. Yet this is still news to many people. His program consists of a mainly vegan diet, exercise and meditation focused on breathing techniques. The changes seen with this program are so powerful that improvements in heart health and symptoms are seen as quickly as two weeks from the beginning of the program. The benefits don't stop there.

A 2010 report from the USDA showed that 36 percent of American adults have blood pressure higher than normal. Thirty-four percent have blood pressure high enough to be diagnosed as hypertension and require medications. Together that is 70 percent or 150 million Americans who suffer blood pressure symptoms. If we suffer with high blood pressure we are seven times more likely to have a stroke, four times more likely to have a heart attack and five times more likely to die of congestive heart failure. We know that the same lifestyle changes that reverse heart disease can lower blood pressure in up to 75 percent of those of us who suffer with hypertension. Not only that, but studies show that over 50 percent of us can completely discontinue blood pressure medication by adopting these changes. When is the last time your doctor sat you down to talk about getting you *off* your medications?

Cancer

It's the second leading cause of premature death in the U.S. We've been at war with cancer for over 40 years, dumping untold hundreds of billions of dollars into research and treatments. This does not account for the man-hours involved or the false hopes and dreams that cancer research generates. The truth is that cancer drugs only save the lives of 2 to three percent of patients.

The number of deaths from cancer continues to rise every single year. These statistics should show us that this phenomenon is not genetic and we are certainly not winning the war.

Let us set aside obesity, diabetes, and heart disease for just a second. The fact that every year more and more people die of cancer should be all the evidence we need as a nation to prove that what we are doing with are bodies is wrong. That the trust we place in the modern medical establishment is wrong and that if we continue to do the same thing without change these numbers will continue to go higher. I fully understand that this is a touchy subject, but it's vital to understand what is really happening in order for us to adopt change.

Let's start with breast cancer to really illustrate this point.

We know that Japanese women have some of the lowest rates of breast cancer in the world. We know that when Japanese women immigrate to the U.S and adopt a typical western diet, their breast cancer rates go up. In Japan, women eat more vegetables, eat less meat, and consume less alcohol while getting more exercise. We also know wealthy Japanese women who eat more meat and animal-based products have a breast cancer rate eight times higher than the poorer women who cannot afford it. We know that breast cancer risk is doubled for women who are 45 pounds or more overweight. These striking correlations are all I personally need to tell me that lifestyle is the most important factor when it comes to cancer.

Facts: The same company that earns millions of dollars a year selling a cancer-causing herbicide also sells the most popular cancer therapy drug, Tamoxifen, and funds National Breast Cancer Awareness Month. I wouldn't be surprised if you are buying the pink ribbons from them as well.*

After college, I learned that one of my friends had become a

* This started as a cynical joke to prove a point about how corrupt these companies are but, as it turns out you may be buying the ribbons from them as well. You'll have to do your own research. Start by researching Imperial Chemical Industries and Breast Cancer Awareness Month to see what you get.

cancer researcher. I semi-jokingly sent him an email saying that his efforts were wasted as many of us already know how to cure cancer. I received no response. But we do know how to cure cancer. Don't get it in the first place. Is prevention not a treatment? Going back to breast cancer, the evidence proves that lowering consumption of animal products lowers your chance of getting breast cancer. We also know that women who walk at least five hours per week can cut their breast cancer risk by up to 15 percent and this is regardless of genetics. More hours walking per week decreases the risk factor even further. The "Long Island Breast Cancer Study Project" showed that exercising 10 hours per week lowered breast cancer risk up to 30 percent! Every time we put something into our mouths we decide the fate of our health. Every time we decide to exercise or not we decide the fate of our health.

For example, lung cancer is the most common cancer from which people die. Studies show that people who eat high amounts of colored vegetables regularly have a 60-percent reduction in lung cancer rates. Therefore it's not surprising that time and time again we come back to the fact that what we put into our bodies and what we do with our bodies influence our health.

The most common cancer in men is prostate cancer. There is an overwhelming body of evidence that shows prostate cancer is highly connected to dairy consumption. This is especially so when you look at the science that proves that men who consume soy milk instead of dairy have a 70-percent reduction in prostate cancer rates. We also know that soy products protect against prostate cancer. That is why there is such a staggering decrease in cancer rates when we cut out a cancer causing agent like dairy and substitute it with a cancer protective food like soy. The math is simple.

We have already discussed the risks of animal products with many different types of disease. This could not be more apparent with colon cancer. The risk of getting colon cancer for people who eat meat just once a week is significantly higher than for people who eat no meat. This ratio exponentially increases as meat consumption per week increases.

Facts: Dioxin can be considered to be one of the most toxic chemicals known to man. It is extremely carcinogenic. Estimates show that up to 95 percent of human dioxin exposure comes from eating red meat, fish, and dairy products.

In the end, it cannot be stressed enough that our lifestyles are intimately connected to whether we will get cancer. Prevention has to be the main treatment for the second leading cause of death in our nation. To further emphasize this, a massive multinational, multi-agency report conducted by the World Cancer Research Fund and the American Institute for Cancer Research was issued in 1997, analyzing scientific research done by thousands of other researchers over the years. It concluded that…

Sixty to 70 percent of all cancers can be prevented by staying physically active, not smoking, eating a mainly plant-based diet and reducing the intake of refined and processed carbohydrates.

Compare these statistics to the 2 to 3 percent cure rate of our beloved drugs.

Chapter 4

Other Hindrances to Your Health

We know that most major diseases are caused by or made worse by obesity. Being overweight, which is 60 percent of the United States, causes a severe risk not only to our health, but also to our economy, our lifestyles, and our families. This creates fad diets and magic pills that steal our money and confuse us even more. Most people who write diet books are out for a buck. Many of these authors have no formal training, no education in health. And what they write about has no science to back it up. Everything written here has come from doctors or scientists, many of whom have spent their careers helping people become healthy again without simply pushing drugs on them. The information that has already been presented can just about save your life and allow you to be strong again, giving you the opportunity to be healthy on your own.

As we have seen, one of the major steps is to lower or eliminate our consumption of animal products. The fact that we do not see high rates of any of the diseases such as heart disease, diabetes, or cancer in people who do not eat meat should help to encourage and motivate you. However, this is a big step for many of us, including me. So, while we try to eat less meat let's look at some other things we can do to make those little changes toward better health.

Ice cream is not allowed in my house. Not because it's bad for you (which it is) but because if it's there, I will eat the entire bucket. And I'm not just talking about those little pints of Ben & Jerry's®. I'll eat a half-gallon if no one is looking. Many people feel the same way about sodas, chips, chocolate; all

Checking Labels

I have a favorite 100-percent whole-wheat biscuit that is great for a snack. One day I turned over the box just to see what was in it and I found MSG. Funny enough, it is only certain flavors from this company that have MSG, so I switched. It is vital that we read lists of ingredients in our food.

the good stuff. With 60 percent of Americans overweight, there has to be something more going on. I would hate to think that all those people think a Big Mac with fries and a soda is OK to eat! Most of us know this is not true. So, what's happening to us? There are two major problems.

The first is actually quite simple. It is called HFCS. This stands for High Fructose Corn Syrup. HFCS is found in most things we love to eat. Its major role is in sodas but it can be found in anything sweet and savory, from breads to condiments. Anything that comes in a box, bag, can, bottle, or freezer section can have HFCS. This is because it is sweeter than sugar and can be produced even more cheaply.

I want everyone to go get their diet-, low-fat salad dressing, mustards, ketchups, BBQ sauces, etc., and turn them over — you probably have a product that has HFCS in it. This is the truest with "diet" and low-fat foods. They take out the fat and add sugar so you'll still eat it. This has been written about exhaustively but for those of you who don't know why it is bad for you and your weight, here it is.

HFCS is a highly processed substance. It is so processed that the body doesn't recognize it as sugar. This is a problem because we have a connection between our stomachs and small intestines to our brains. When we eat food, these connections say, "OK, that's enough, no more food." When we eat HFCS, this connection isn't stimulated. This allows us to eat more before our brain gets the signal from the other foods that enough is enough. We've just eaten more than we probably would have. Scientific evidence also shows that HFCS increases cholesterol levels. So one of the simplest things you can do to start improving your health is to avoid HFCS in your foods.

The second area of concern is a little more difficult. This involves any refined and processed foods. Again, anything in a box, bag, can, freezer section, or bottle has more than likely been processed. This is done so the "food" does not spoil. It is a fact that the healthiest parts of foods are the ones that spoil more quickly. Therefore by eating things from supermarket shelves, you are consuming highly refined and processed foods devoid of any nutrition. One need only to turn the product over to read in the list of ingredients that vitamins and minerals have been added back in, but usually not in a form the body can process. Now we get none of the nutrients and all of the empty calories, making us fat.

Facts: Over 60 percent of products on supermarket shelves contain genetically modified or engineered ingredients. We don't know what these things will do to our bodies in the long run. Without solid evidence, I can at least promise they won't make us any healthier.

There's another dirty little secret to refined foods, especially when it comes to simple carbohydrates: sugars. It's the reason that when I'm tired or grumpy or stressed I'll shove the vegetables to the side and saddle up to a bacon cheese burger with fries dipped in ranch topped off with a tub of peanut butter chocolate ice cream before bed.

These processed foods contain an overabundance of refined sugars. These refined carbohydrates spike our blood level of serotonin. Serotonin is what Prozac™ and similar antidepressant drugs work on. Serotonin keeps our mood even, makes us happy, feeling good and energetic. When we eat all these breads, pastas, pastries, cookies, candies, chips, French fries, ice creams, and so on, we're stimulating the release of this brain chemical, making us happy. This is where the term "comfort foods" probably came from. These foods can end a bad day in a good way, help us through a stressful week and get us over challenging times in our lives.

The truth is that many of us feel stress every day and there is always something going on that we could feel better about. These foods act like drugs to our bodies and we, as a nation, are absolutely addicted to them. When sugar and refined foods spike our serotonin levels, there's always the inevitable crash. Many of us know this because we start to snack on things although we have recently eaten. Most of us know that we are not hungry and don't need any more food. Unfortunately, for most, the will power is just not there.

I cannot tell you how many times I had a nice, healthy dinner planned for after work, only to come home tired and throw that frozen pizza into the oven. *Tomorrow though, tomorrow I'll eat a better dinner. Right?* Right enough, that serotonin spike will be well gone in the morning and I'll be my regular self. That is of course if we were just talking about serotonin.

There's also fat, particularly the saturated fat you find in meat, milk, and milk products like butter, cream, and cheese – the type of fat in many snack foods like chips; the oil used to deep-fry French fries. Most baked goods and breads have oils and butters in them that contain saturated fats. We know these saturated fats trigger an increase in dopamine in the brain. Dopamine is one of the principle neurotransmitters that make us feel warm and cozy all over. This is the same chemical that marijuana and other drugs work on. When these products are eaten regularly in the diet, dopamine causes the same reaction the drugs do: a tolerance. This means it takes more of the substance — here it is saturated fat — to get the same response. On the other hand it means that the same amount of food does not give us the same feeling as it once did. We need more. We continue eating even if full. We eat too much. We make bad choices.

So now we have spikes in serotonin and dopamine making us feel good. But, after the fact, we crash, feeling even lower. And at the same time, we've built a tolerance to these chemicals, leading to cravings and dependencies. Therefore it's fair to say that refined and processed foods, especially with saturated fats and refined sugars, act as drugs do. We have seen this in our nation, a nation of obese and sick people, a nation of slaves to food.

Of course this is compounded by the fact that when we do get sick, all we have to do is go to the doctor and get a pill so we can continue doing the same thing. I have heard many people argue that they would rather live life and be happy than try to embrace the changes necessary to be healthy. Trust me when I say that having chronic pain, heart disease, cancer, or the plethora of autoimmune diseases that come with poor choices in life is not living at all.

Chapter 5

Your Gut

Many people do not understand alternative medicine. It can sometimes be difficult to explain to people what I do. This is the example that I give to illustrate the difference in how practitioners of alternative medicine view the body and treat our patients. One of the top-selling and most-taken over-the-counter medications is an antacid. It's safe, simple, and it works fast. Your stomach hurts; you take a pill. If your indigestion gets worse or starts to become more regular you go to your doctor and they will give you a prescription antacid. You now have to take this on an ongoing basis or else you will continue to suffer.

From my standpoint your stomach is not supposed to have pain when you eat. Indigestion and acid reflux are symptoms that something deeper is not working properly. Instead of giving you a pill to mask these symptoms I ask the question, "Why do you have heartburn in the first place?" The question is simple and the answer is what's needed to truly make you healthy once again, just like you used to be. This is how medicine should be practiced. To answer these questions, we first need to have a little basic knowledge of the digestive tract.

Food and air are the two things the body always needs to live. Our bodies are constantly breaking down and repairing themselves from the food we put in. It's the fuel that powers us as humans, and it shocks me how overlooked the importance of nutrition is in modern medicine. Our bodies don't overlook it, though. At least 80 percent of doctor visits are GI (gastrointestinal) related. Heartburn, acid reflux, gut pain, gas, bloating, constipation, and diarrhea are the most common complaints. These symptoms are our body telling us that the fuel we're putting in is wrong. This is just the beginning, though. Left unchecked, these gut-related problems can lead to more serious issues with our health. We have to look at several main areas to understand what causes some of the diseases in humans stemming from our gut and what we put into it.

Toxins

We absolutely know that toxins in our environment cause all types of problems and diseases. But what if those toxins were being produced inside us? Now our bodies must process external environmental toxins and internal toxic chemicals, a double assault to the system. If we eat the wrong types of food or if our digestive systems are slow and weak, food will begin to rot. The bacteria and yeast inside our guts are doing the rotting and — just like when we ferment beer or wine — toxic chemicals are created as by-products. In this example, it's alcohol. However, there are many types of bacteria and yeast inside us and they release various toxic chemicals as food is rotted. Initially, this will cause gas and bloating, a symptom that tells us this is going on.

Some of these toxins alter the way the intestines work, forcing you to retain water and become constipated. Sometimes the intestines become irritated by the toxins, pushing water the other way, creating loose stools and diarrhea as the body tries to clear everything out. These symptoms of gas, bloating, heartburn, constipation, loose stools, and cramping tell us there is sometime wrong with our digestive tract. These are the initial signs and left uncorrected can lead to more serious health problems. These toxins trigger and over stimulate our immune systems, as well as create inflammation in our guts and in our bodies.

Weight Stalling

The liver is one of the main players in the weight game. Signals from the liver can control fat metabolism. Fat in the body is one of the main storage units for internal and external toxins that we encounter daily. In the end, the body does everything it can to protect itself from damage. If the liver is dealing with the toxins that are coming from our gut, it will not send the signals our body needs to start breaking down fat because that would create an even more toxic environment. This is just one aspect of stubborn fat. The intestines must be processing food appropriately and eliminating quickly. We must be eating healthy foods that do not create this toxic environment.

Our immune system

Autoimmune diseases are on the rise. I see so many patients who come in for one thing and at the same time have Crohn's, ulcerative colitis, diverticulitis, asthma, allergies, rheumatoid arthritis, hypo/hyper-thyroid and other intestinal and systemic problems. The first question that needs to be asked is, "Does it make sense for our bodies to attack themselves?" No, and the fact that autoimmune diseases are on the rise shows us the trend is a product of something we're doing to ourselves, not a product of genetics.

The second question is "What triggers our bodies to attack themselves?" For the most part, modern medicine doesn't know. In alternative medicine, the reason is actually very simple. Except for the small percentage of viral or genetic causes, these abnormal responses of our immune system are caused by two factors either independently or in combination: stress (see Chapter 6) and diet. There are numerous correlations between diet, how our bodies digest food, and autoimmune diseases. The exact mechanism has yet to be discovered, but the pathway is quite obvious.

Seventy percent of our immune system is centered around our intestines. Because our intestines bring the outside world in and are directly connected with the bloodstream, it's highly important that the wrong things don't get in. If we put the wrong kinds of food in, such as refined and processed foods, excessive amounts of animal products, dairy — or if we let the previously mentioned toxins build up — this can trigger a response from our immune system. Just like anything else that alters the way our body functions, this can cause permanent changes if nothing is done to correct it.

This example always seems to surprise people and it's deceptively simple. If our blood pressure is too high for too long, eventually it will get stuck and we'll be hypertensive. If our blood cholesterol is too high for too long, eventually over time it will get stuck and we'll have chronic high cholesterol. If our blood sugar is too high for too long, it will get stuck and we'll develop type 2 diabetes.

Our bodies adapt to change, for better or for worse. Therefore if our immune system is triggered, day in and day out, by the wrong foods and the subsequent toxins being created, sooner or later that process will get stuck and the body will start to attack itself. This is how we trigger the genes that create disease. We trigger these genes through our actions and the decisions we make every day, every time we put something into our mouths.

Inflammation

It's a well-known fact that inflammation in the gut can spread to the rest of the body. What we eat can either lower and reduce the inflammation response in the body or increase it. The inflammation caused by what we eat affects our entire body, but there is one major disease that will eventually affect most of us. Let us explore one more piece to the heart disease puzzle.

We've been on an anti-cholesterol campaign for over 40 years. Many foods on the shelf boast of having no cholesterol. Cereal companies have fronted major advertising campaigns to let people know their cereals contain high amounts of fiber. We know that fiber can reduce cholesterol and reducing cholesterol helps to reduce the risk of heart disease. Yet, rates of heart disease have been steadily rising to this very day. The cholesterol in our blood may eventually kill us, but it is not the cholesterol that starts us down the road to heart disease.

Heart Disease Puzzle Piece #2 Inflammation in the gut can spread to our blood vessels, creating inflammation and damage. This inflammation, especially coupled with high blood pressure, causes serious damage to our blood vessels. This is where cholesterol starts to play its part. It's cholesterol that's used to repair the damage to our arteries. With time, this process is repeated over and over and starts to create thick patches of fat called plaques. These plaques, combined with inflammation and a hardening of the arteries, define heart disease and lead to heart attack and stroke. This is why changing diet to eliminate cholesterol is not enough and usually ends with you taking serious, toxic drugs to force cholesterol levels down. The inflammation must be reduced for our blood vessels to be healthy and this starts with what we eat.

Food Intolerances

This seems to be a growing problem in our society. I have more and more patients in my practice reporting that they cannot eat certain foods. In my mind this seems counterintuitive. Why, as humans, would we have a problem eating food the Earth provides for us? I remember a couple of instances when I was teaching and had foreign students in my class who were surprised at this. In their countries, they'd never heard of such a thing.

There are several pathways our bodies take to handle allergens. Some, such as anaphylactic shock, are life-threatening. Some, such as hay fever and seasonal allergies are downright annoying. And some, like food intolerances, can be happening under the radar without us even knowing. This can go on for years until this slight reaction finally triggers a bigger problem in the body. For example, let's look at what we call a wheat allergy.

Being allergic to wheat is actually a disease. It's called celiac disease and is serious because, after a while, the patient is unable to digest food because of the damage caused by the allergy. What we hear about in the news and popular culture is actually a gluten intolerance. Gluten is a protein from wheat (allergies are caused by proteins). In a normal person's gut, this protein is too big to pass into the bloodstream and trigger an allergic reaction. But add in the years of toxins and inflammation from the previous section, and we get a situation in which the previously benign gluten protein can slip into our blood and create a low-grade allergic response. I have known people who have cleaned up their diets, reduced the inflammation in their guts, and found themselves able to eat moderate amounts of wheat once again.

In addition, many people with food intolerances and gastrointestinal problems have also been shown to have an improper balance of healthy vs. unhealthy intestinal flora. Although there are many contributors to healthy intestinal flora, for our purposes we're talking about bacteria. Beneficial bacteria are crucial for us to digest food properly. Just like in the movies, there is the good and the bad. They always co-exist, and usually the good keeps the bad in check. Unfortunately, because of the rampant and liberal use of antibiotics, many people have killed off their intestinal bacteria and again, just like in the movies, the bad guys always bounce back first.

Now, with the intestines populated with bad bacteria, other bacteria and yeast can come in and take over the fermenting of food inside you — instead of helping you to digest. This problem also leads to everything we've talked about previously, such as inflammation and the buildup and absorption of toxins into the bloodstream. This concept must be explored if you've taken long and/or multiple rounds of antibiotics, and especially if you've had odd symptoms or developed something new within one year of taking antibiotics. This can be a big issue in people who have trouble losing weight. This is one aspect of what we call "slow digestion" but is really the improper balance of intestinal flora.

Replacing the Good Guys

Eating fermented foods such as miso, sauerkraut, tempeh, kombucha, and yogurt on a daily basis can help replace the good bacteria inside you. If you do not eat these foods then you can buy a pro-biotic supplement from the health food store. Make sure that it is in the refrigerated section and that it has a guarantee that the cultures are live. Six to eight weeks will typically be enough time to fix things. It's crucial that diet is also changed to lower the amount of refined sugars and flours, because this can be counterproductive, feeding the bad bacteria.

Chronic pain? Fatigue? Gastrointestinal problems? Chronic colds and flu? Allergies or asthma? One of the most important aspects of changing your diet for the better is to identify any possible food intolerances so your immune system gets a break. Reduce the inflammation and pave a solid road for better health. There will be a list of common foods that trigger the immune system in appendix B as well as information on how to figure out whether or not you are sensitive in Chapter 7.

What's interesting is that the same nutrition that prevents heart disease can reduce inflammation in your joints. The same dietary patterns that prevent diabetes also prevent autoimmune disease. The same lifestyle that prevents cancer also prevents obesity and can lower blood pressure. All these major diseases are linked to what we put into ourselves, every meal, every day.

Chapter 6

The Mind

I have tried to make the previous chapters as simple and concise as possible. If you're like me however, you're probably getting sick and tired of reading about how we are making ourselves sick and tired. I always receive the same response from my audiences. Therefore when I lecture, as in this book, I promise to have a bright and happy ending. Bear with me as we cover one more aspect of your body, an aspect that's frequently overlooked, even in writings from some of the most comprehensive doctors out there. It astonishes me that this information is not more prevalent and available to people and that our doctors almost completely ignore this topic.

The mind and the body are so intimately connected that it would be completely unethical and unprofessional not to have a chapter in here about the mind. The brain and nervous system are responsible for controlling digestion as well as willpower to choose to eat well or not. Out of all the information I've previously mentioned, this topic is always the one that surprises people the most. This is most likely because it is complicated and can be technical. I'll try my best to have it make sense.

Stress is said to account for up to 80 percent of general practitioner visits. This seems like an awfully high number but, as we'll see, stress can manifest itself in many ways and affect many systems of the body.

First, let me define stress. In basic psychology, stress is defined as the inability to cope with situations encountered in daily living. I like this simple explanation because it makes it very personal for all of us. What stresses me will be different from what stresses you. For example, I have lived in Los Angeles most of my life. I think of traffic as downtime — time to relax and listen to some music or chat with a friend. It's me-time. I know that many people do not feel the same way.

What this points out is that we are the ones causing our own stress. This is very important, because we actually have the choice of whether certain daily situations get to us. It is our decision, and what we'll see is that we can change the way we react to stressful events. Although I like this definition, I think it is too limited. A broader view must include more than just "stress."

It's estimated that more than 70 percent of people who develop serious illness, usually chronic, have had a high level of stress or a traumatic experience within one year preceding their very first symptom. This brings other factors into the picture: a death in the family, a divorce, car accident, loss of a job, and so on. This is a big key for many people who suffer with symptoms for which doctors cannot find causes, such as fatigue, headaches, and digestive complaints. These can then turn into more serious disorders such as fibromyalgia, chronic fatigue, IBS, migraines, depression, anxiety, and other somatoform (functional) disorders. These are essentially disorders of stress and we will see how they evolve. Simply, if you suffer from something and you've been from doctor to doctor and no one knows what's going on, it's a big indication that stress or trauma is involved.

Finally, to get the complete picture, we will define stress to include any emotion that controls you and you cannot control. Sadness, grief, and regret are one category. Anger and frustration; fear; worry and pensiveness (over-thinking); lack of joy in one's life and/or lack of connection with other people — if any of these are a consistent, day-to-day feeling for you, then it's possible that these can be a source of stress on your body. From this point forward, to make things simple, I'll just use the word "stress," but please keep in mind that all of the above can exert the same changes in your body. These changes are separated into two main categories: neurological changes and chemical changes.

Neurological effects of stress are the fastest-felt and most noticeable. In the long run, they can cause extensive damage to the body.

Dr. Herbert Benson, a Harvard medical cardiologist became curious one day about why the American public was suffering from increased rates of heart disease, despite the fact that we'd been on an anti-cholesterol campaign for so long. In his research, he found that it was not the cholesterol but high blood pressure that was the major influence in heart disease. Now the search was on for what caused high blood pressure (hypertension). Unfortunately, even to this day, if you look at a medical diagnosis book you will see that 80 percent of hypertension is idiopathic. Idiopathic means that our medical professionals don't know what causes it. After years of research, this cardiologist figured it out: it was stress.

One of the first things that stress does is trigger the sympathetic (fight or flight) nervous system. This raises heart rate, blood pressure — you might even get a little sweaty. This is how lie-detector tests work. The problem that Benson found is that stress can be real (money problems, family/relationship issues) or imagined. If you were hooked up to diagnostic machines and I had you close your eyes and imagine something that really made you angry or something that frustrated you, your blood pressure and heart rate would go up. Just from imagining a scenario!

Many of my patients and people I've met fall into this category. We worry, over-analyze and over-think about situations that happened in the past or have not even happened at all. This worry causes stress, and triggers the same response as if it were really happening. Just like everything else in the body if this reaction is going on all day long, everyday, eventually the body will get stuck and your blood pressure will stay high. It will stay high even on the weekends and even if you go on vacation. This high blood pressure coupled with the inflammation coming from the gut starts you down the path

Heartburn, Acid Reflux, and Ulcers

Medical professionals used to think that some of these conditions, especially ulcers, were cause by bacteria called H Pylori. We know now that H Pylori are part of normal flora in our body. However, under the stress response the PH in our stomach changes, allowing these bacteria to overpopulate. This is when it starts to cause a reaction that leads to ulcers. It's no coincidence we see high rates of ulcers in Type A people. In addition to this we know that overeating, eating foods you are sensitive to as well as alcohol add fuel to the fire when it comes to ulcers, heartburn and acid reflux, typically in combination.

toward heart disease, heart attack, and stroke.

What stresses me out is that this Harvard cardiologist went on to conduct research studies and publish books on the subject in the 1970’s. Yet, when you go to your doctor with headaches, fatigue, heartburn, bowel problems, insomnia, and especially high blood pressure — instead of taking a good hard look at the underlying causes such as stress and diet — your doctor will give you a pill. That pill does nothing to treat the reason your body isn't functioning correctly. It's a pill that doesn't fix you but merely masks the symptoms of disease, forcing your body into a "healthy" state, and leaving the real problems to never be addressed.

For example, stress causes muscles to become slightly more tense and tight. Year after year, these muscles get tighter and tighter and will eventually produce those knots we're all so familiar with. Those knots are the most common cause of headaches, thereby making stress the No. 1 cause of headaches. This is just another way of your body telling you something deeper is wrong. But do we listen?

Only one nervous system works appropriately at a time. While the fight-or-flight system is active, the rest-and-digest (parasympathetic) system slows down. Now, keep in mind the last section on your gut: inflammation, immune responses, and the buildup of toxins? This is where a lot of it starts. If the rest-and-digest system turns off, your intestines start to slow down. Eventually the food we eat, even healthy food, starts to rot, creating an environment that leads to disease. Gas, bloating, constipation, loose stools/diarrhea, and heartburn are some of the first symptoms telling you your body is not happy. Again, even if you're eating healthily, under this process those good-for-you fruits and vegetables can turn into toxins and inflammation.

Then there are the chemical affects of stress, which are longer-lasting and cause more diffuse changes in the body. Although many chemicals are released when we experience stress, the major player is cortisol. Cortisol comes from our adrenal glands, which sit on top of our kidneys, and it has several functions in the body.

Cortisol triggers the liver to do two things. The first is to increase production of cholesterol, which raises our blood levels. Combined with the fact that animal products and meat also trigger the liver to raise cholesterol levels, this starts to pave the way to heart disease, despite how much cholesterol you are actually eating. The fact that stress can raise cholesterol levels is often overlooked and should always be addressed.

The second affect cortisol has on the liver is that it stimulates a reaction called gluconeogenesis. That's a fancy word meaning to create sugar from nothing. This is another function of the liver that most people are not aware of. In times of stress or physical exertion, the liver can take other fuels such as proteins and turn them into sugar. So that hamburger, fries, and soda are bad enough, but add them together by going back to a stressful job or eating on the run and you get a double whammy. Now we know that stress raises blood pressure, blood cholesterol, and blood sugar, which are all major causes of disease. This can be a major stumbling block for you if you're trying to eat healthily, lose weight, and lower cholesterol and/or blood pressure.

Do you feel like you get sick frequently or have chronic sinus or other recurrent infections? Cortisol dampens your immune system. Once again, this becomes a double-edged sword. On one side, we have cortisol knocking out the immune system. On the other, we have a slow digestive process (from the flight-or-fight reaction), creating the buildup of toxins and inflammation which are stimulating the immune system. This clash leads to confusion and can be the missing link as to why our bodies start to attack themselves and why autoimmune disorders are on the rise. It's no wonder so many chronic diseases can be linked to stress.

Are you in pain? Do you have good days and bad days? Is the pain worse in the morning or is it worse at night? Quite simply, if you had something that was totally physical, then you would be in pain all the time. Every time you moved or did some activity, it would get worse. If you have good days and bad days, then it's fairly safe to say that your pain is coming from inflammation in the joints, muscles, or tissues of the body. In fact, if you have any symptom that comes and goes, you must look at stress or inflammation as a trigger. The reason for this is that when stress triggers the release of cortisol, this chemical also interferes with the way your body deals with inflammation. You may already know that doctors give cortisone shots for chronic pain sufferers. What this does is simply disrupt the inflammation cycle, and in the end it makes everything worse.

One would think that quieting this cycle would be good and reduce pain. But it's inflammation that comes in to heal and regenerate the body. If it is interrupted and disturbed, then chronic inflammatory diseases ensue.

I spent several years working with surgeons and it was quite obvious that the patients who were more stressed about the surgery and how it impacted their lives did not heal as fast. Many of my patients already know that stress makes their pain worse. Because stress releases cortisol and at the same time facilitates more inflammation from the gut, it is vital that you give stress a good hard look if you suffer from chronic inflammatory diseases.

Hormone changes. Although it is the brain that regulates the release of our hormones, it's the liver that breaks down and eliminates them from our body so that they can fluctuate properly. This applies more for women because without the proper ebb and flow of hormones, female bodies do not work correctly. Regular menstrual cycles need the liver to work at its best in order to maintain healthy levels of hormones. If the liver is busy producing cholesterol, making sugar, and dealing with inflammation and toxicity, it has a hard time performing its job. This leads to hormone changes that cause PMS, infertility, and low libido. However, hormonal problems are just the tip of the iceberg. It's the liver that breaks down estrogen to be eliminated from the body. If the liver is busy and estrogen is only partially broken down, it forms very toxic metabolites (by-products). It's no surprise, then, to see that many chronic diseases and autoimmune diseases — especially when they involve inflammation — affect women, at least three to one, over men.

If this is stressing you out, don't worry, this is the last major effect of stress and, as I said before, there's a happy ending to this tale: there are ways of managing stress without winning the lottery or quitting your job.

Stress — through many factors both chemical and involving the nervous system — causes a decrease in our serotonin reserves. Serotonin keeps us happy, energetic and feeling good. Serotonin is created from amino acids broken down from proteins in our diet. Unfortunately, under stress, your digestive system is not working well and cannot replace the serotonin being used. Soon we start to feel low and tired, grumpy and irritable. That's when sugary and fatty foods start to call to us. Without proper levels of serotonin our willpower starts to dissolve and that salad turns into pizza and going to the gym or for a walk turns into "tomorrow." We start to crave anything that will make us feel good again: food, sex, alcohol, drugs, anything.

If this vicious cycle is not dealt with properly and our serotonin levels go lower, the mind and body suffer even more. Depression can set in. That's when we go to a doctor feeling moody and blue maybe even fatigued, and we're given an antidepressant. But we're not depressed…are we? No, it's just low serotonin levels caused by trauma, long periods of stress, or a poor diet. Most likely a combination of more than one of these.

Without proper serotonin levels, it becomes more and more difficult to control our thoughts. That's why some of us develop anxiety, which is simply defined as chronic worry. Worrying, or over-thinking, is also a form of stress on the body and sets up this vicious cycle. Many cases of depression and anxiety are just the end result of chronic and enduring stress. Many doctors will prescribe a six-months-to-a-year "trial" of antidepressants, but a good majority of my patients have been on them for many years. These drugs don't treat the root of the problem, which is the stress causing a serotonin deficiency. Certain breathing techniques that I'll talk about later have been proven to reverse the stress response, allowing the body a chance to heal and correct the imbalances that were started so long ago. It's a shame how many people come into my office with depression or anxiety. I ask if their doctors have shown them how to breathe properly. The overwhelming answer is no.

Last but certainly not least, research shows that about 40 percent of Americans suffer from insomnia. Regardless of what my patients come to see me with, I have seen at least 60 percent of them check the box next to insomnia. Some have trouble falling asleep. Bad sleeping habits, overstimulation from TV, and a restless mind can all keep you up at night. Some people wake up several times during the night, and some wake up too early without enough sleep. It's not surprising to see that insomnia is also linked to what we eat, and to stress.

Melatonin is the chemical that regulates normal sleep patterns. What's interesting is that melatonin is intimately connected to serotonin. The more serotonin we have, the more melatonin — because serotonin gets converted into this sleep chemical. The less serotonin, the less melatonin, and sleep problems ensue. Low serotonin and melatonin play a large role in people who can't "shut off" their minds or cannot sleep the entire night through.

Stress is only one aspect of your not being as healthy as you want to be. As we've seen, it's a very real reaction in the body that affects many of us, day in and day out. It's the most overlooked cause of disease, which is frightening considering that stress is somehow involved in many people who suffer with a chronic disease.

Luckily, just like adopting a better diet, there are things you can do to overcome stress and regain control over your mind. Like changes to diet, this also requires you to take back responsibility for your health and stop pawning it off on the pharmaceutical companies. Please see Appendix C for learning how to control the stress response.

Chapter 7

Baby Steps to a Healthier You

Being six-foot-two I am naturally a big boy. By the time I hit 23 years of age, I was pushing 250 pounds, which might have been a little too big. One day, after catching a glimpse of my backside in a double mirror, I was shocked into action. I went out, bought running shoes and shorts, and hit the streets. I made it two city blocks before I was huffing and puffing and admittedly a little dizzy. So instead, I started walking. Being a health professional I knew what to do and how; I just had to do it. Eight months later, I had gotten down to a beautiful 185 pounds, which is my perfect body weight. Then somewhere around age 30, I got lazy again. They say time heals all. This must include memories of me being fat. By the time I knew anything was going on, I was back up to 230 pounds! So it was back to the streets and six months later back down to 185 pounds. I have watched my mom do the same thing, one of my sisters, my brother, and many of my patients, let alone all the people we see on TV. By now, every single one of us should know that diets do not work. If you see anything advertised as a miracle diet or diet pill or anything else that does not require you to take action…run!

Instead, what 60 percent of Americans need is the knowledge of how their bodies work and how foods affect them. That's hopefully what you've received from this book.

The second thing we need to understand is that being a healthy weight and being healthy in general is a lifelong plan. To be completely and absolutely vibrant, we have to make good choices every day and make sure we take care of ourselves on an ongoing basis. This involves lifestyle changes. But, as we know, jumping into something and radically changing your life almost never works out in the long run. That's why it's so important to make small changes very slowly over months and years to eventually achieve your goals. Obviously, if you suffer from a particular illness you may want to start embodying more of this information faster. For most of us though, it is healthier and wiser to do it more slowly to obtain longer-lasting results.

First Things First: Nutrition

We have seen undeniable proof that the over-consumption of animal products and dairy are seriously detrimental to health. Let's start slowly. Know that dairy is unfavorable and that we should view it as a treat. I love cheese. It's one of my favorite things on this planet. However, I know the truth. When I do eat it, I make sure that I see it like we should see cookies, candy and other sweets: it should be special. If you suffer from any autoimmune disease, heart disease, asthma, allergies, gastrointestinal problems, osteoporosis, or kidney disease, dairy should be eliminated from your diet or eaten in extremely small amounts and rarely.

Figure out how many times a week (or day) you eat dairy products and try to cut one-third of it from your diet per week. For example, if you eat dairy every other day, about four days a week? — try eating it only three days a week. Do this for a month. When you are successful with this, then next month try cutting it by half for another month or even two. Remember, the slower the changes, the more consistent they can be. Once you do something for a couple of months it becomes automatic, a habit. Once successful with half, start aiming lower, to a point at which dairy consumption is only for special occasions.

When you start this journey, also take care to increase dark green leafy vegetables such as spinach, kale, collard greens, broccoli, and Brussels sprouts, as well as nuts and seeds (especially almonds) to get the calcium you need in your diet. Good milk substitutes are soy, almond, hemp, and rice, but be careful and read the label to make sure they are not loaded with hydrogenated/ partially hydrogenated oils and sugar.

Set goals and keep track. Many of us are so busy that we don't remember what we had for breakfast, let alone a week's worth of food. Keep a log. This takes two minutes if done after every meal. Write down what you ate and drank during that meal. It does not have to be complicated.

For example: Lunch, Friday the 18th, turkey sandwich with cheese, small salad, small bag of potato chips, iced tea with sugar. We see here this is a carbohydrate-heavy meal that includes both meat and cheese. So next time we can try for just the turkey sandwich with a relish, mustard, or hot sauce instead of the cheese and a serving of nuts or seeds instead of the potato chips.

In the beginning, a log will be helpful, but soon enough thinking about what you are actually eating will come automatically.

Meat and Meat Products

This includes red meat, pork, chicken and other poultry, eggs, milk, cheese and other dairy such as creams and butter. And yes, even fish and seafood are meat. As I mentioned earlier, scientific evidence and research done on people around the world shows us that eating meat negatively affects our health. At the same time, our bodies are designed to process animal protein. Therefore I argue for moderation. There is too much proof that vegetarians are healthier than meat-eaters in almost all aspects of disease. Do I really think this will convince most people to become vegetarians? No, and really nor will I. However, if you are sick, especially with high cholesterol, high blood pressure, heart disease, cancer, an autoimmune disorder, or if you have a family history of these and this scares you, you might want to consider cutting as much animal products and meat out of your diet as possible. Remember, there are several very prominent doctors out there who have absolutely proven that heart disease can be reversed without surgery through eliminating all animal products from your diet.

Starting slowly, I ask people to try to limit animal products to one meal a day. This is a good start. I try to practice eating animal products one meal a day, every other day. Sometimes I am successful, sometimes not, but at least I am conscious, knowledgeable, and trying. You can do the same.

Without all the meat and dairy, the body is able to heal itself faster so the more ill you are, the more you'll want to cut these out. The end goal based on science (and being reasonable with regard to our society) would be eating meat and meat products for only one meal two to three times a week, much like what we would have done as hunters and gatherers, back when our bodies were developing.

This is about the time that people get confused and start to panic. “So what do we eat?” In trying to keep this simple I will go over a little information about other foods and if you're serious about being healthy, you will have to see Appendix E for healthy-living cookbooks.

Vegetables, Vegetables and More Vegetables

After I say this to people I always hear, "I know, I know, I know" or "But I don't like vegetables."

Well, of course you don’t like vegetables. Especially when your brain, taste buds, and hormones have been trained and conditioned on bacon cheese burgers, pepperoni pizzas, and pasta carbonara for years on end. Seriously, bacon and cream sauce? I wouldn’t eat broccoli either. But we have too. It was in my early 20s when I was trying to lose weight that I discovered vegetables. I didn’t like them either. I’ll never forget one night in particular when I was invited to a new girlfriend’s house for dinner. She was very happy to have me over for a meal that she prepared and so was I. I sat down at the dinner table hungry and interested to see what she'd made. The first thing she served was a beautiful salad with a stunning variety of vegetables and a homemade salad dressing. Halfway though my salad I asked if I could help her with anything else and told her that I was excited about having what she made for dinner. She replied a little hesitantly “this is dinner.” That being over 10 years ago, my memory is a little fuzzy, but I'm pretty sure this scenario fueled our first disagreement and ended with me going to get takeout.

Nowadays, I am perfectly content having a salad for a meal,

which I eat for most of my lunches during the workweek. I also try to make sure that three to four dinners a week are salads or at least all-vegetable dishes. Starting slowly, you must first make sure that every meal has some vegetable. Many of us have weak digestion after years of processed foods. Going straight into raw vegetables might be tough at first so try steaming or lightly sautéing your vegetables to begin with. When you are ready, try creating at least one meal a day that is a combination of cooked and uncooked vegetables with some type of whole grain or legumes (beans). The combinations are endless and if you are not kitchen savvy then it might be best to pick up a couple of vegetarian cookbooks and start experimenting. Try to make it an activity for yourself and the family. Have fun and explore the possibilities food can offer. There are thousands of combinations and flavor options. Remember, especially when working with salads and raw vegetables, that many of the calories, preservatives, additives, HFCS, and other things we don't want are often in the sauces and dressings. These are very easy to make on your own and that also allows you to expand your flavor horizons.

Fruit

An apple a day keeps the doctor away…really? Yes! Apples eaten raw and in their whole form have many protective affects on the body. Apples lower blood pressure and cholesterol. They also dredge the body of harmful heavy metals that we encounter in our daily environment that can lead to age-related diseases. And we're just talking about apples! In the interest of keeping this book as short as possible, just know that a healthy diet should include a variety of fresh fruits and berries. Like apples, all fruits and berries have some sort of beneficial effect on the body. They are full of nutrients the body needs to function properly. They contain enzymes that vegetables do not have. These enzymes can help us digest other foods better and support a healthy digestive tract which, as we have seen, is vital to good health. Berries and dark-colored fruits have very special antioxidants found virtually nowhere else that protect the body from damage -- damage from our polluted environment and damage from the internal inflammation and toxicity we generate. They are also some of the strongest agents to protect us from cancer. Some, such as tomatoes, have chemicals that protect the heart; some, like pineapple, have chemicals that reduce the inflammation associated with arthritis. The list goes on and on so EAT YOUR FRUITS AND VEGETABLES!

Is eating organic necessary? In a word, yes. If your fruits and vegetables don't say they're organically grown, then they've been sprayed with herbicides, fungicides, and pesticides. We absolutely know that these are cancerous and toxic to the body. However, only some fruits and vegetables retain these chemicals all the way to your kitchen. Unless you want to walk into the grocery store with a botanic chemistry book then it is just easier to buy organic. Almost everywhere in the U.S. you can find these items and the trend is getting stronger. Demand organic and the supply will get stronger, lowering the prices and saving your health.

Fruit Juice

Almost all the fruit juices in the store are nothing but non-carbonated soda. As a child, I always had my glass of orange juice in the morning and my juice box for lunch. These days I see so many people drinking fruit juice during a meal, probably thinking they're being healthy while everyone else drinks soda. Read the label. How many calories and how much sugar is in your favorite juice? Most likely the same as soda. Now look at the nutrients. Are there any? Look at the ingredients and see that many times the nutrients have been added, turning that orange juice into vitamin sugar water. Then, so these "juices" can sit on the shelf, they've been pasteurized to death, destroying most of the beneficial nutrients you thought you were getting. Lastly, one of the greatest benefits of eating whole fruit is the great amount of healthy fiber in the skins and peels. So, if you're not freshly juicing the fruit yourself don't waste your time.

Grains

For years now, there has been a lot of controversy, misinformation, and unscientific commentary on grains, i.e. carbohydrates. Most of this completely ignorant information has come from these low-carb diet fads. These scams have no science to back up any health claims and go against thousands of years of carbohydrates being the staple of almost every society on our planet. Yes, there are very real reasons why cutting back on them helps you lose weight, but the truth of the matter is that it's not a sustainable diet. Many people gain back the weight they lost after a couple of years, and often they gain even more weight then when they started. If you were to cut back on carbs (as refined products) and eat more fruits and vegetables, then I would congratulate you, but the low-carb diets promote meat in place of the carbs. We now know this is the exact opposite of what we want and is worse for you in the long run because it promotes disease.

Carbohydrates are an extremely important part of our diet. The problem with carbohydrates is that most people simply don't know which ones are good for you and which ones promote ill health. We have to know this. Most societies around the world survive very healthily on grains. Our bodies' primary source of energy is carbohydrates. Unless we're staving to death, our brains only run on sugars. Sugars are not only healthy but absolutely necessary for us. Fifty to 60 percent of our diets should be healthy carbs. The facts are relatively easy to understand. Carbohydrates: fruit, breads, root vegetables, pastas, cereals, rice, pastry, cookies, cakes, and sugars are not created equal. What causes detrimental health risks such as diabetes is how fast those carbohydrates are broken down and absorbed into our blood. This is the glycemic index (GI) of a particular carbohydrate. The higher the GI, the faster it absorbs, the faster you blood sugar spikes and the more insulin is released into the blood. It's the sugar spike and increased levels of insulin that promote disease. Other factors such as the amount of fiber or fat the food has also changes the GI. There are many good online resources for finding out the GI of different carbs, however it is important not to get bogged down here. All the other foods in the meal can change the GI of a particular carb, so saying this is a good carb versus bad carb is really not enough.

HEART DISEASE PUZZLE PIECE #3 High GI foods (glycemic index) spike blood sugar. High blood sugar damages arterial walls. On top of this, it's the high blood sugar that triggers an increased production of insulin. We've known for awhile that a decreased sensitivity to insulin is the primary factor in type 2 diabetes. But there's mounting evidence that shows that high insulin levels can also damage arterial walls. Cholesterol then starts to attach and patch the damage caused by the high blood sugar and high levels of insulin. Plaques start to form.

The easiest thing to remember is if your carbohydrates come from vegetables and whole grains that have not been completely processed, they're OK. The processing is important though. By this day and age all of us should know that refined white flour and sugar and the products made from them are fairly useless as a food substance. They are stripped of all their fiber and nutrients and then bleached white for appearance. They have nothing our bodies need, just empty calories. They spike our blood sugar and cause disease. The rabbit hole only gets deeper, though, as certain companies are out for a buck.

In his book *Eating Well for Optimum Health*, Dr. Weil exposes a very interesting fact. If we look at the GI of white bread then at the GI of whole-grain bread we see that they're about the same. This is because the whole grains are processed into a superfine powder used to make the dough. When the grains are this fine, they absorb just as fast into the body even if the package says it is 100-percent whole-grain. Stone-ground or coarse-ground grains would be preferable, and the more fiber the better.
At the very least, you should start reading labels and knowing what's inside your food.

Baby steps. Start cutting back on anything out of a box, bag, bottle, freezer section, or can and start to work on making your shopping basket as close to 70-percent fruit and vegetable as possible. Start to pick up vegetarian, low-GI or anti-inflammatory cookbooks, and try experimenting with them a couple of times a week and growing from there.

I love bread too, but try cutting back on the breads, pastries, cookies, chips, etc. And when you do buy them, find the coarse- and stone-ground 100-percent whole-grain versions that have lots of fiber and no hydrogenated or partially hydrogenated oils. When you do go all out and eat breads, pastas or potatoes, add lots of vegetables to the dish because this will lower the GI of the whole meal. Add a little olive oil. Olive oil is a healthy fat and fats lower the GI of carbs.

Many of you have heard about the Mediterranean diet which is loaded with the things we love including breads and pastas (carbs!), but at the same time is supposed to be heart-healthy. The breads are typically served with olive oil and vinegar. Vinegar as well as olive oil also lowers the GI of carbohydrates. The pasta's are loaded with vegetables, not meat, and cheese is used sparingly.

I have traveled the Mediterranean for months on end and have eaten in many places. I remember the meal at one restaurant, quite specifically. This place was known for their lasagna and I was excited. The first thing I noticed was that out of the many lasagnas to choose from, there was only one with meat, which I ordered. The bread that's usually at our tables first came with the meal, which happened time and time again in most restaurants. I always ate less bread in these countries because of when it was served. As an American, I'd say the lasagna came in an extremely small dish with heaps of vegetables, very little meat and, to my taste, a disappointingly small amount of cheese. Only a small side salad was offered. In the end, the people in these countries eat smaller portions with more vegetables, report lower stress levels, and get way more exercise than we do.

Fats and Oils

In the previous sections, we saw that dietary cholesterol by itself is not responsible for causing heart disease. In fact, the right dietary fat is healthy and necessary for our body to function properly. But like carbohydrates, not all fats are created equal. The information below can guide you in one of the easiest aspects for changing your life to enjoy better health. Let's look at the different types of fats.

Saturated fats are bad. They're found in animal meats and dairy products like milk, creams, cheese, and butter. These fats promote inflammation in the body and blood vessels, raise blood cholesterol, and disrupt the clotting factors of the blood, making your blood thicker and more difficult for your heart to push. This increases your risk for strokes, heart disease, and heart attack. Read the label. If a product contains saturated fat, it will still raise your blood cholesterol even if the product says *no or low cholesterol!*

Trans fats have been all over the news lately and we know they're bad. Luckily, food manufacturers have slowly stopped using them. However, there are fats out there that do not come from nature and react negatively in the body. These are the hydrogenated and partially hydrogenated oils that are in so many snack foods and fried foods. These oils have been transformed into something not usable by the body for healthy cell function. These fats are super-heated with highly reactive metals like nickel, transforming the molecular shape. When most fats and oils are heated too much they turn rancid and become carcinogenic. Last time I checked, our nation did not need any more cancer-causing substances in our food, nor have I ever read that we needed more nickel in our diet.

One of these strange fats is the margarine (fake butter) family. Although it's a fat, it doesn't raise cholesterol levels because the body doesn't know what to do with it. So for years, it has been touted as a healthy alternative to butter. Like genetically modified foods (GMO), there's no concrete evidence showing that margarines are dangerous, but these synthetic oils in my opinion are a closer relative to plastic than food. And the hydrogenated and partially hydrogenated oils used in so many things *do* have science to support the fact that they cause inflammation and negative changes to our blood vessels, making the cardiovascular system work harder. Turn over your foods and read the labels. It could not be easier to start avoiding these unhealthy, unnatural substances in our lives.

Monounsaturated and polyunsaturated fats reduce inflammation, raise good cholesterol, and lower bad cholesterol. They promote healthy blood clotting and scientific evidence is showing that they can protect the heart and blood vessels against heart disease. These types of fats are also starting to be shown to be good for the skin, complexion, brain, mood, and your joints. These good fats are found in whole grains, dark green leafy vegetables, cold water fish, some fruits like avocados, nuts, seeds, and certain oils especially olive oil, hemp seed oil, walnut oil, and flax seed oil. By increasing healthy fats and decreasing unhealthy fats you can start to make a serious difference in your health. Here's how.

Omega 3 is the healthy fat found in foods from the paragraph above and is highly beneficial to your body. Omega 6 is a not so healthy fat. Omega 6 promotes inflammation, which makes everything from arthritis to heart disease worse. Our bodies need both because this is how we function, but it needs both in a certain ratio. That ratio is about one to four (omega 3 to 6). The typical American diet has an incredibly high ratio of damaging omega 6 and extremely low amounts of beneficial omega 3. The main reason why omega 3 is lower in our diet is because of modern farming practices. When wild animals eat their natural wild diet, their fat and meat contain more omega 3. When "factory-farmed animals" are fed foods to fatten them up quicker, the ratio switches to the animal having more pro-inflammatory omega 6. For example, it is estimated that you would have to eat twenty of today's factory-farmed eggs to get the same omega 3 as one free-range chicken egg. What's causing this?

To get an animal as fat as possible as fast as possible it's usually fed grains; more specifically corn. Corn has a ratio of one to 46 (omega 3 to 6) making it *highly* inflammatory. The cows are fed corn, the chickens are fed corn, the pigs are fed corn, and in some places in the U.S. the farmed salmon have been raised to eat corn. This is one of the major reasons that our diets, which are so high in animal products, contribute to the ever-increasing rates of heart disease, hypertension, heart attack, and stroke. Unfortunately it does not stop with just our meat. Remember, corn is used to fatten up animals and that applies to humans, as well.

Take a couple of food items from your cupboard and your fridge.

Start reading the backs. You'll find in most things ingredients made from corn. Corn starch, corn flour, corn oil and high-fructose corn syrup all combine with the corn our animals are eating to add up to a lot of inflammation and a lot of diseased, overweight, and sick people. So here is a tip. While it's extremely beneficial to start cutting down on your consumption of animal products, it's equally vital to start eating free-range, naturally fed animals. Now, at least when you do eat animal protein, it will be higher in the healthy anti-inflammatory omega 3. Further down the road of better health is to buy organic meat. If the package does not say organic then the animal is most likely shot up with drugs, antibiotics, hormones, steroids and who knows what else. All these chemicals get stored in the flesh and milk of the animals and enter our bodies when we eat them. I do not know about you but that does not sound very appetizing to me.

CHEATING

Although excess protein is harmful to our bodies, the most damage is done by the inflammation caused by eating animals fed foods high in Omega 6. While you try to start lowering your consumption of meat and animal products, a great way to instantly improve your health is to switch to organic free-range **grass-fed** or **natural-fed** animals. It's all about money. If it's not labeled like this, then all the farmers have to do is truck out the corn and dump it in the middle of a field

EXERCISE

If you were to type in the following quote into a search engine you would find articles from the National Institute of Health and the Centers for Disease Control and Prevention. As well, there will be current TV reports and a multitude of "new" stories and articles that say just about the same thing.* I have been using this quote since at least 2007 when I came across it in a medical book that adorns many doctors' shelves (probably collecting dust).

> Lack of exercise is the second leading cause of premature death; second to smoking.

* Sometimes the quotes say that lack of exercise is the third leading cause of death. Nonetheless, it is of paramount importance.

The human body was meant to move. All our internal organ functions, our nervous systems, our brains, and our blood flow depend on us constantly moving. Yet we sit at the breakfast table before we sit in the car to work, where we sit all day, and then sit in the car to come home, and sit at the dinner table, before we sit in front of the TV, before we lie down for bed…and we wonder why our nation is getting fatter and sicker.

The science is in. We need to move to stay healthy. We need to move to stay pain-free.

In the end I ask the question: is waking up in pain, struggling in the morning before our drugs kick in to survive until lunch, when we need to take the next round of drugs to survive the rest of the day -- all the while having tummy troubles, depression, and pain, unable to truly live our lives and do the things we want to do (especially if we're retired and finally free!) -- worth 45 minutes a day?

Because that's all it takes. Here's the absolute bare minimum to keep the body functioning well. Remember that exercise is so important to the body, it can actually help prevent cancer!

- 30 to 45 minutes of brisk walking five times per week.
- 30 minutes of cardio once per week.
- 20 minutes of resistance training twice per week.

The walking alone can be life-saving. Walking regulates almost all of our internal organ functions. It protects against cancer, facilitates proper digestion, and can double brain levels of serotonin helping with mood and sleep. That, and it supports core strength along the spine, helping people with back problems.

Cardiovascular ("cardio") exercise is essential for heart and lung function. It's also necessary if you're trying to lose weight, as it can increase your metabolism. This type of exercise is anything that gets the heart beating faster than it beats when at rest. Most of us remember Sylvester Stallone in *Rocky* skipping rope. Skipping rope is an incredible cardio workout. Jogging, swimming, climbing up stairs, riding a bike, and so on, are all good types of cardio exercise. For many, especially those who live with chronic pain, it's important to find a professional to help you start this.

Resistance training involves lifting weight or using your own body weight to strengthen the muscles. Aside from diet, increasing muscle tone is the No. 1 factor in reversing or preventing diabetes. It's also equally important, if not more so, in maintaining strong bones and preventing osteoporosis (the weakening of bones as we age). I know that many who read this will imagine big grunting men with no neck who can't scratch their own backs, but this is not the case. This could be as simple as climbing stairs for the legs and butt muscles, grabbing a gallon of water in each hand and doing some arm and shoulder work, push-ups, crunches, and whatever uses the muscles till they get tired.

Here's a little disclaimer. If you suffer from a serious illness, especially heart problems, or have chronic pain or spinal disorders, then it will be necessary to obtain help from a qualified professional. The first person I would go to would be a physical therapist. But, as in all professions, there are good physical therapists and bad ones. I would look for them in pain-management centers, sports rehabilitation centers, or those working for heart surgeons to rehabilitate people after heart surgery. You can also try personal trainers. My suggestion would be to find trainers in private practice before you hire one in a gym. Regardless, they should know what you're talking about. If you find a personal trainer and tell them that you have spondylolisthesis and cannot walk for more than 10 minutes without having to sit down, he or she should know what you're talking about. If a trainer doesn't understand your personal medical condition, then keep looking. Again, as I'm trying to keep this book simple, you'll have do your own research and find a good book or DVD on this issue but, that's what all of this is about anyway: taking back *your* health.

Team Work

Plain and simple. The reason our species has become the dominate force on this planet is because of teamwork. I know too many people who have tried, but failed, to embrace the changes outlined in this book. These are people who sit down at the dinner tables and stare at all the food that is killing them, eating their tofu-and-spout sandwiches while their families gorge. This does not have to be the case, but one person in a family cannot do this alone. These changes will save all of our lives, and if you live in a family, the whole family will have to participate. This does not have to be a chore, though. These changes can be fun as a family starts to cook together, exercise together, and find healthy hobbies. These changes can help bring a family closer while at the same time making every family member healthier. This might take a while and can be a real struggle especially for kids who have been living on refined and processed foods, but it's possible to accomplish. Let children help you cook and don't mention the word "healthy" or the phrase "good for you." Just pick a healthy recipe, let them help you cook, and they'll be excited to try something and will have no idea. If you live alone, then there are many online and local support groups for whatever you're trying to do. I cannot say it enough, keep looking, keep trying, and work together.

Food Intolerances and the Challenge Test:

Genetic predisposition, heritage, medications, inflammation because of stress and poor food choices along with environmental toxins can all add up and lead to food sensitivities over time. These may start when we're young or old, and can change over a lifetime. Because of all of these factors, many people nowadays are sensitive to one or more food groups, which is a shame.

What does "sensitive" mean? -- simply that a certain food or family of foods triggers a low-grade immune response and can also cause a chronic inflammatory state in the body. How do we know? Certain types of doctors such as naturopathic doctors (NDs), dieticians, nutritionists, proactive MDs, doctors of osteopathy (DOs), doctors of acupuncture and Oriental medicine (DAOMs) and a few others can send out for blood tests that cost several hundred dollars and tend not to be specific. To give an example: typical tests for gluten intolerance only test for the one major protein in wheat, while other proteins can cause the same reaction in the body.

The easiest and least costly way is to do it yourself.

Eliminate from your diet for at least three weeks all inflammatory foods -- dairy, high-GI foods, all or most animal products, and most foods from a box, bag, can, bottle, and freezer section. In addition to a change in diet, a 24-hour clear broth or juice fast is done every seven days during those three weeks. See Appendix D for instructions on juice and broth fasting.

I usually recommend three weeks because when the inflammation starts to settle and healthy foods are being put in, the body will send a signal to start dumping the toxins it was storing. This can cause a secondary inflammatory response and quite possibly induce flu- and cold-like symptoms. This is typically called a "healing response" or, more often, a "healing crisis." When I do this, I typically have some bowel troubles for the first couple of days as my body starts to really clean things out. I also usually feel very tired for those first couple of days, as well. For that reason, it's important to start on a Friday or another day that will allow you to rest as much as needed for a couple of days.

Now, the whole point of this book is to make this information simple to assimilate as well as easy, or rather, easier to implement into one's life. Sitting here writing this, I know that many people will not do this unless they're sick and tired of being sick and tired. For myself, I would need a good deal of motivation to do this for three weeks. So, if your medical problems are minor and have not been going on for too long, you can try a simpler -- albeit not as comprehensive -- route.

Pick one category of foods from the food-intolerance list (Appendix B) plus all dairy and eliminate them from the diet for at least three weeks. It will always be a food group plus dairy. At the end of the three weeks, eat a large meal primarily with that food group (no dairy). To give you an example; the nightshade family (potatoes, tomatoes, all peppers and chilies and eggplant) has a chemical that in some people can worsen the inflammation related to arthritis. For three weeks, eliminate all foods from the nightshade family and at the end, have a large meal consisting of only nightshades.

Gas, bloating, diarrhea, heartburn, fatigue, an elevated heart rate within 20 to 30 minutes of eating, insomnia and increases in pain or the symptoms of your disease within the first 24 hours are all good signs that you are sensitive to what you just tested.

Then, give yourself a break and in a week or so test another category.

The only downside to this is that many people are sensitive to several things and trying one at a time might not get the most pronounced reactions. Of course, if you're suffering with an illness or a lot of pain then the three weeks with the fasting will be necessary and if you are trying to test against an autoimmune disorder then a month will be necessary. After all is said and done, it's a good idea to do a 24-hour fast every couple of weeks to give the body a break and allow it to clean itself out. Remember, our bodies weren't meant to process food all day long, day after day, let alone handle all the processed gunk that's packaged and sold to us as food.

Lastly, because this book was kept intentionally short, I cannot stress enough that this is just the beginning. It's my hope and my intention that what you have read here will motivate you to do further reading into how our bodies work and why we have gone down such a disastrous path of ill health. Please see Appendix E for more outstanding books by some of our nations leading doctors, scientists and authors.

In the end, your health is ultimately up to you.

I hope that just knowing this information will help you start to make informed decisions about what you do with your life. I always tell my patients that even if they just try, they're doing good for their bodies.

Try getting rid of some of the junk, and little by little start adding the healthy things to your life. Soon these little changes here and there will start to add up to big changes that help all of us live longer, more vibrant lives. In the many years I've been in practice, I've personally witnessed miracles. In that time, I've heard even more stories from my patients about the miracles they say they've witnessed. I believe it's never too late for change.

Never give up!

Appendix A

Have you tried everything?

If you have tried changing your diet in a way similar to what's presented here -- if you've tried exercise consistently for several months and you've tried stress management and still don't feel well, then you might want to read on.

There is evidence that the overgrowth of a yeast called candida can cause a wide variety of symptoms and illnesses. Several factors lead to such overgrowth in the body. If the mix of symptoms and signs sounds like you, then it might be time to find a doctor who is open to hearing what you have to say. Because candida is a natural part of our flora, it's difficult to test whether you actually have an overgrowth. Here are the signs and symptoms, along with circumstances that can lead to overgrowths.

Section 1 ~ Circumstances

- Repeated or prolonged antibiotic use.
- Hormonal changes, such as pregnancy or using a birth-control pill.
- Steroid use (typically prescribed for pain, autoimmune disorders, various chronic diseases).
- Diabetes and/or a diet high in sugars and processed foods.
- Repeated exposure to an infected partner.
- High levels of stress.

Section 2 ~ Symptoms

- Fatigue.
- Headaches.
- Depression.
- Digestive complaints (gas, bloating, constipation, loose stools).

- Recurrent vaginal, urinary, or bladder infections.
- Chronic sinusitis/rhinitis.
- Asthma.
- Recurrent colds and/or flu.
- Food intolerances.
- Chemical sensitivities.
- Infertility (all other factors have been ruled out).

If you have one or more from each category, have been from doctor to doctor trying to find out what's wrong with you, or have been diagnosed with a functional (somatoform) disorder and/or a disorder diagnosed by excluding everything else (such as IBS, chronic fatigue and fibromyalgia), then you might want to consider a systemic yeast infection as part of the problem.

If you have a child with learning problems such as ADD/ADHD, psychological, behavioral and/or nervous-system problems who also has a history of recurrent ear infections and antibiotic use, then it's also recommended that you find a doctor open to discussing the possibility of a systemic yeast infection. See appendix E for more reading.

Appendix B

Immune System Triggers

It is entirely possible that you are sensitive to a variety of different foods or chemicals in food. Therefore, the following is not necessarily a comprehensive list, as you could be sensitive to just about anything. This list comprises the most common types of foods that over stimulate our immune systems and create inflammation in the gut. Anyone suffering from any chronic inflammatory disease, chronic autoimmune disease, skin disease, or emotional disorders, should follow the challenge diet outlined in Chapter 7, going though one item or category at a time. This could take up to six months to complete but is well worth it to end your suffering. Look for small changes because many times it's a combination of foods in the categories below that cause a problem and not just a single one.

1. Any and all food colorings, additives and preservatives. Do your research and you'll see that many supposedly "safe" food colorings and additives come with a list of symptoms associated with that particular coloring and/or additive. I would highly encourage everyone reading this not to test against these and simply eliminate them completely and forever from your diet.

2. Monosodium Glutamate (MSG). Even if the package says "No added MSG," it does not mean there's no MSG. MSG comes from natural sources and can be in food without the manufacturers having to label it. Therefore also keep an eye out and avoid anything "hydrolyzed," "autolyzed," or "textured."

3. Dairy, which includes butter, cream, milk, cheese, and dairy products hidden in products on the supermarket shelf like milk solids, milk powder, whey, whey powder, and anything with the word casein in it such as sodium caseinate.

4. Wheat, anything made from wheat flour and anything that contains gluten. This is such a big deal that nowadays many

products must label whether food contains gluten or is made from wheat.

5. Corn, corn flour, corn starch, corn oil, and high-fructose corn syrup.

6. Fructose and fructan. Evidence is starting to mount that about 20 percent of the population is sensitive to fructose in what's called fructose malabsorption. This is most likely because of the rampant use of high-fructose corn syrup and wheat flour in our foods making us sensitive to what is a naturally occurring sugar found in many things including what it's named for, fruit. The USDA has a database on fruits and vegetables high in fructose, but some of the more common ones are: artichokes, asparagus, leeks, onions, wheat including most beers, breads, cakes, biscuits, breakfast cereals, pies, pastas, pizzas, and some noodles, apples, pears, honey, sucrose, most dried fruits and most fruit juices. This is a crucial group to test, especially if you suffer from any digestive complaints, insomnia, depression, or fatigue. Fructose can limit the amount of tryptophan we absorb from our food, and tryptophan is the building block of serotonin (happy mood, good digestion) and melatonin (sleep).

7. The nightshade family. This is especially important for people who suffer with arthritis. Tobacco, tomatoes, potatoes, all peppers and chilies, and eggplant.

8. Eggs.

9. Sulfite(s) in wine and potato chips as sodium bisulfite or potassium bisulfite.

10. Nitrites in most cured and dried meats. This chemical stops bacterial growth and gives meat that pretty dark red color. It reacts with the protein in meat if it is heated and can form toxic nitrosamines that are known carcinogens.

11. Tyramine in cheese and most foods that are pickled, aged, smoked, or fermented such as soy sauce, miso, teriyaki; also in fava beans, green beans, snow peas, avocados, bananas,

pineapple, eggplant, figs, red plums, raspberries, peanuts, brazil nuts, coconuts, yeast, and unfortunately, chocolate. In sensitive people, this chemical can cause elevated blood pressure and migraines.

12. Citrus fruits and anything that contains citric acid (which is in a lot of foods as a preservative).

13. Then some odd ones like bananas and strawberries.

Appendix C

Undoing Stress

There are two main aspects of managing stress.

The first is mental which includes stress triggers (boss, money, traffic, lost luggage, etc.) and what I call the stress habit. This is where there have been long periods of stress or a trauma that create very real neural connections in the brain.

The second is the subsequent nervous system and chemical changes in the body. The latter is easier to control so let's start there.

Find a quiet place. Find the pulse in your neck by finding the lump on your throat halfway between your sternum and jaw. Then roll your fingers over to the right side of your throat between your throat and that big neck muscle. Sit for a second and feel how fast your heart is beating. When you have a good idea how fast it is ticking take the biggest, deepest breath you can and hold it for five to 10 seconds. Don't count but again focus and pay attention to how fast your heart is beating. Your heart rate should slow down significantly. What you could not notice was that your blood pressure also dropped. By taking a deep breath and holding it you stimulated the parasympathetic (rest and digest) nervous system which, as we learned, is the opposite of the stress response.

Don't worry, you won't have to spend the day holding your breath. Through practice, you'll teach your body how to do this without holding your breath. The most important point is that you breathe with your belly. Most people who suffer stress, depression, anxiety, and insomnia don't know how to breathe properly. Lying flat on your back, put one hand on your chest and one on your belly. Start taking nice, deep, full breaths in and out. Only the hand on your belly should be moving. Some people get this right off the bat. For others, it can take a couple of days and some real focus. Once you're able to breathe with your belly lying flat, try to take this practice with you in the car, at work, and pretty much everywhere else. This is how we're supposed to be breathing. This type of breathing stimulates the vagus nerve which controls heart rate, blood pressure, and all of our internal organ functions. The vagus nerve handles the vast majority of what we call the rest-and-digest nervous system. Read the next section through, then try it yourself.

Find a quiet spot and a chair or get into a comfortable position on the floor if you are able. Sitting upright in an erect but not rigid position close your eyes and take a nice, deep, belly breath in…hold it for just a second…then exhale and feel all of your muscles start to relax and let go. Now, focus on your toes. Feel any tension you might be holding in your feet. Tell yourself to relax your feet and "let go." From here, focus on your ankles, relaxing, releasing and letting go. Do this all the way up your body. Engage your calves, knees, thighs, low back, then circle around to your belly, back again to the spine, working your way very slowly up your spine, focusing on and relaxing all those muscles that support you all day, and letting go of all the tension you hold on to. From here, work your way down your arms, elbows, forearms, wrists, and fingers, again making sure to relax all the individual muscles, telling yourself to let go of anything you might be holding onto. From your hands you come back up to the neck, relaxing your neck and putting your shoulders down. This is where so many people hold so much tension.

You may find that you have to tell yourself to put your shoulders down a couple of times. That's OK. Keep trying. Once the shoulders are down and relaxed, work up your neck over the top of your head and pay attention to your forehead. Release the forehead muscles letting them relax, then all those little tiny muscles around your eyes. Relax your jaw letting it drop a little and letting go of any tension you might be holding onto in your jaw. Just let it go. Once again take a nice, big, belly breath in… hold it for a second…then as you exhale, imagine that from the top of your head all the way to the tips of your toes, all your muscles are relaxed and released. Also, as you exhale, imagine any tension you might still be holding onto disappearing with the air that you're breathing out.

This is called progressive muscle relaxation. It is a fantastic way to de-stress. Most of us put stress away in our muscles and in the long run this can cause problems. This is also a great way to start a sitting meditation session. On the off-chance that I can't sleep or wake up in the middle of the night, I'll start a progressive muscle relaxation and usually not even make it to my shoulders before I'm out again.

The next section is the actual meditation, which is the key to breaking those neural connections (the habits) and resetting your nervous system to a state of relaxation. If you have trouble with the next section -- if the mind just keeps chattering away by itself -- then start the muscle relaxation again, beginning with your toes and following the same pattern we just did.

What you are about to learn is called mindfulness. It is not thinking about the past and what used to be or what you could have done better. It is not worrying about the future and things that haven't happened yet. It's simply being in the present moment in which you are truly alive and in which life is actually going on. Being in the present moment can change your life for the better and, quite possibly, the lives of the people around you as you start to realize what's important and what is not. Being present and connected with life and the people around us is the ultimate in living, and being able to do this will be the cure for stress and the undoing of trauma. However, like everything else in this book it is not a quick fix and it takes practice. Mindfulness is a tool, a skill that has to be learned and practiced just like anything else.

OK. Still in your quiet spot, having just gone through the progressive muscle relaxation, I want you to focus on a place in which you can physically feel your breath. This could be your nose, the back of your nose, your throat or belly, but somewhere that you can physically feel air move in and out. If you feel a sensation like an ache or a pain, simply acknowledge what you feel, let it go and focus on your breath. If you hear a noise, acknowledge it for what it is -- noise -- let it go, and go right back to your breath. Most importantly, you will have thoughts -- you might have hundreds of thoughts, that's OK. As long as you are trying you are doing a good job for your body. When you have a thought simply acknowledge it -- “Hmmm, I’m thinking” -- let it go and go back to your breathing. In the beginning, your mind will continually come up with things to think about. Again, if it is really noisy in there, then start over with the progressive muscle relaxation.

Baby steps. This is a learning process. You are breaking old habits and forming new ones and learning a new skill set. This takes time. Research shows that it takes 45 to 60 days to undo neural connections and reform new, healthier ones. This must be practiced for 10 to 15 minutes every day for this to happen. Start slowly. Aim for three times per week. After a couple of weeks, try four and so on until you find 10 minutes of quiet time every day for 45 consecutive days. Watch over time as life seems to become more peaceful. Notice how things that used to trigger you now seem silly. This simple technique is quite amazing, once learned.

If you suffer from anxiety and find it difficult to sit still, then try other practices that employ meditation with some sort of activity such as yoga, tai chi, or qigong. These practices are so powerful they're becoming quite popular and can be found in most cities and towns. I've seen many people get off their medications by learning these techniques developed by a Harvard cardiologist. Careful, though. You should always consult the prescribing doctor before you stop any medications. If your doctor is not open to these practices despite how much scientific evidence there is to support them then I would have to say it's time for a new doctor. Keep trying; this is about your health, not your doctor’s.

Appendix D

Juice and Broth Fasting

It's important for us to give our digestive tracts a break once and a while, especially since our modern diet is so loaded with artificial this and preservative that; all the sugar, all the fat, let alone the pesticides, herbicides, and fungicides, and the fact that many of us overeat. Because of all of this toxicity, I recommend that if you're suffering from something, you try to do a 24-hour fast every week for the first month or two. The more serious the disorder, the more months you'll want to do this. This is also applicable to -- and very helpful for -- those who want to do the challenge diet. If you're healthy, then once or twice per month is great to keep your body clean. Some say a good fast to clean everything out can take anywhere from seven days to two weeks. But my fast protocol is meant for the average, working, and most likely sick individual. Therefore, we do shorter but more consistent fasting. If you're able to do two or three days, then by all means give it a go.

Healing Soup

3 cloves garlic

2 carrots

2 tablespoons chopped cilantro

2 tablespoons chopped parsley

½ large onion

2 tablespoons fresh ginger

3 quarts vegetable stock, organic, yeast-free, low sodium, no MSG

1 small yellow squash

½ beet with green tops

1 small head broccoli

3 stalks celery

1 tablespoon organic, first cold pressed, olive oil

Some people might be sensitive to the high amounts of sulfur in the garlic and onions so you can modify this accordingly but all the ingredients are in there for a reason. If you're testing against the nightshade family then substitute the vegetable broth for water as many of the premade broths contain bell peppers.

The garlic cloves can go in whole. Chop the carrots, onion, ginger, squash, beet, broccoli, and celery into pieces a little bigger than throwing dice, to allow you to strain it more easily when you're finished. Bring this soup to a boil and then quickly reduce to a simmer for 30 minutes. Strain all the solids out and squeeze to get as much broth as possible.* Have a cup or two every three to four hours to stave off the hunger pangs. Three times a day, with the broth, take a 1,000 mg capsule omega 3 supplement of high quality (these will usually be 3 times more expensive than the rest). After the 24-hour fast, I highly suggest you do not go back to your normal diet but try to introduce, little by little, at least some of the knowledge we've covered in the previous sections.

Juice Fasting

In my mind, there is nothing better for your health then regular juice fasts. However, buying the juices from the store is fairly useless. To sit on the shelf in the refrigerator section, they've been heat-pasteurized, killing many beneficial ingredients. On top of this, these juices are usually high in pear and apple juice and/or sugar, so you will actually drink them. This pasteurized, high-fructose concoction defeats the purpose of juice fasting. If you are serious about your health and undertaking regular juice fasts, then it will be necessary to invest in a machine to do it yourself. I highly recommend not getting the cheap juicers that use blades to chop and pulverize the veggies. A good machine will run $400 to $600 and will use a technology that squeezes the vegetables. These are usually called "slow juicers." It's not in my interest to sell you anything, as I believe good health advice should be

*I don't like to waste food so I'll take the strained vegetables, put them into another pot, add more broth and make a soup to eat the next day. I usually remove the ginger just before eating; it can be difficult to digest

available to anyone interested. So you'll have to do your own research. I advise seeing if friends or family owns one of these high-quality juicers and asking to borrow it for a month or so before making the investment. Please see Appendix E for further reading on juicing.

Appendix E

Further Reading

In my mind there is no chronic disease or illness that doesn't have an answer in one or more of the following books. If just one can be life-saving, then imagine what the whole lot would do for you, your health, your family, and our world. Now is the time to take the next step and continue down your road to being happy and healthy.

In alphabetical order of title:

Dr. Dean Ornish's Program for Reversing Heart Disease: The Only System Scientifically Proven to Reverse Heart Disease Without Drugs or Surgery

Ref. Ornish, D. *Dr. Dean Ornish's Program for Reversing Heart Disease*. New York, NY: Ballantine Books, 1996.

Written by Dean Ornish, MD. Although there have been other doctors who have proven that heart disease can be reversed, Dr. Ornish was one of the first to prove it with scientific research in great enough numbers. This book outlines the facts about heart disease, what causes it, and, most dramatically, not only how it can be stopped but also how it can be reversed! This is a must for anyone who doesn't want to go under the knife, take toxic and deadly medications, or die of a heart attack or stroke. The reason I like this program is because it focuses not only on diet and nutrition but also on stress management, which, as we have seen, is really a key to lowering blood pressure.

Eating Well For Optimum Health: The Essential Guide to Bringing Health and Pleasure Back to Eating

Ref. Weil, A. *Eating Well For Optimum Health*. New York, NY: Alfred A. Knopf, Inc., 2001.

Written by Andrew Weil, MD. Dr. Weil is one of the most famous and best-regarded physicians in the field of alternative and integrative medicine in the U.S. He is the author of many books on diet, nutrition and health. Eating Well For Optimum Health is an easy–to-read and well-written book on how to change your diet to stay healthy and even reverse disease. What makes this a rarity among books on diet is that Dr. Weil firmly believes that eating well does not have to be a sacrifice to one's happiness. He asserts that it's entirely possible to eat well and enjoy your food. He has great stories of people who were left behind by the general medical establishment but were able to beat their diseases through dietary and lifestyle changes. The last portion of the book contains delicious and easy–to-prepare dishes from appetizers to desserts!

Guided Imagery for Self-Healing: An Essential Resource for Anyone Seeking Wellness

Ref. Rossman, ML. *Guided Imagery for Self-Healing*. Tiburon, CA: H J Kramer, 2000.

Written by Martin L. Rossman, MD. This is a wonderful book for people who are dealing with more than just stress in their lives. This is for the millions who have been through traumatic experiences -- or have had trauma and emotional problems passed down through their families to them. Dr. Rossman explores how stress and trauma affect our bodies, and offers more than techniques to alleviate stress – he also covers how to get in touch with the subconscious to find out why we aren't well. This book is definitely for anyone with psycho-emotional problems and/or for people with symptoms that don't add up to an easy diagnosis. This is a must-have if you remember your very first symptom(s) of your disease, starting within a year of a trauma or stressful event. This is also an important book if you've tried making changes in your life and always failed – or if you sabotage yourself in your repeated attempts to adopt a healthier lifestyle.

The Anti-Inflammation Diet and Recipe Book: Protect Yourself and Your Family from Heart Disease, Arthritis, Diabetes, Allergies – and More

Ref. Black, JK. *The Anti-Inflammation Diet and Recipe Book*. Alameda, CA: Hunter House, 2006.

Written by Jessica K. Black, ND. Dr. Black has written a very easy-to-read book that outlines the basic do's and don'ts of eating well. The concept of reducing inflammation through diet is the basis of what everyone is talking about when it comes to preventing disease. With 125 recipes, this is a great book to start with as you try to embrace healthy eating. Not only are the recipes delicious but I also love her liberal use of herbs and spices in place of salt and fats, along with tidbits of information on why these foods are healthy for us. She does have many animal-based recipes but most adhere to a low-animal-protein diet. Definitely a great book to bring into your kitchen.

The China Study: The Most Comprehensive Study of Nutrition Ever Conducted and the Startling Implications for Diet, Weight loss and Long-term Health

Ref. Campbell, TC and Campbell, TM. T*he China Study: Startling Implications for Diet, Weight Loss and Long-Term Health*. Dallas, TX: BenBella Books, 2006.

Written by T. Colin Campbell, PhD, and Thomas M. Campbell II, MD. After 40 years of biomedical research, leading a 27-year laboratory study (one of the longest ever), plus writing hundreds of peer-reviewed scientific articles and obtaining hundreds of thousands of dollars in research funding, Dr. Colin Campbell is one of the greatest pioneers in diet and nutrition research. The China Study, which contains over 750 references, most of them from primary-source research, is the authoritative text quoted by most books to follow it. Almost everything in One Less Excuse is supported by The China Study. The quote from Dr. Dean Ornish on the front cover of the Campbell book sums it up: "…reading it may save your life." This is a nutritional bible.

The Food Revolution: How Your Diet can Help Save Your Life and Our World

Ref. Robbins, J. *The Food Revolution*. Berkeley, CA: Conari Press, 2001.

Written by John Robbins. Mr. Robbins was heir to Baskin-Robbins until he renounced that empire after realizing the devastating effects of junk food on health, the economy, and our planet. John Robbins has written other national best-sellers including *Diet for A New America. The Food Revolution* is a great start for many readers. Mr. Robbins explores not only how diet and nutrition affect our health but how our choices in what we eat affects our environment, and how and why corporate America is keeping us ignorant of the truth. This is a not-to-be-missed book if you want to know why the United States' population continues to get sicker. This is the quote from the back cover and I agree wholeheartedly.

"Carefully researched, eminently readable and starkly accurate, The Food Revolution will change your life. If every patient in every doctor's office read this book, it would revolutionize the health of America." –Neal Barnard, M.D., President, Physicians Committee for Responsible Medicine.

The Everything Juicing Book

Ref. Jacobs, C and Johnson, P. *The Everything Juicing Book.* Avon, MA: Adams Media, 2010.

Written by Carole Jacobs and Patrice Johnson. Carole Jacobs is the former nutrition editor for Shape magazine. She has teamed up with Chef Johnson and a certified dietician, Nicole Cormier, to create a very simple and easy-to-read book for those who have never juiced before. Those new to juicing will find a great deal of information in here as well as recipes that taste great. For those who are looking for a little more in-depth knowledge and more recipes, there is the *Big Book of Juices* written by Natalie Savona. I just like to throw one of everything into my juicer, but the word "delicious" would never be seen anywhere near one of my recipes.

The pH Miracle: Balance Your Diet, Reclaim Your Health

Ref. Young, R. *The pH Miracle: Balance Your Diet, Reclaim Your Health.* New York, NY: Warner Books, Inc, 2002.

Written by Robert Young, PhD, and Shelly Young. This book has a little different view of health-through-nutrition from others. Dr. Young looks at how the foods we eat change the pH of our blood, which leads to tissue damage and subsequent illness. Although Dr. Young focuses on pH instead of inflammation, it turns out that his diet is mostly the same as everything the science supports in other books (although he is a little more strict about grains). I like this book because it does offer a different view of the body and of health, although the end is the same. Change your diet, change your life. In The pH Miracle, you will see the science, hear personal healing stories, and be provided with sample meals, recipes, and supplement advice and well as more information on juicing.

The Relaxation Response

Ref. Benson, H. *The Relaxation Response*. New York, NY: HarperTorch, 2000.

Written by Herbert Benson, MD. This is a shame. This Harvard cardiologist discovered the devastating effects of stress on the body and published this book, which has sold millions of copies. Yet it seems that no one, especially your doctors, has paid attention because medical schools still teach that there is no known cause for high blood pressure in 80 percent of people who suffer with it. The reason this is a shame is because Dr. Benson published this book in 1975! This is a very easy-to-understand book with very simple answers to many of our stress-related questions. The technique taught in this book is similar to what I've presented here and can be a very powerful tool in changing your life. This is a must-have book if there is any stress in your life.

The Yeast Connection Handbook: How Yeasts Can Make You Feel "Sick All Over" and the Steps You Need to Take to Regain Your Health

Ref. Crook, WG. *The Yeast Connection Handbook*. Jackson, TN: Professional Books, Inc, 2002.

Written by William Crook, MD. If Appendix A made you think twice, then this book is the next step to regaining your health. Dr. Crook is an authority on the subject of candida overgrowth and this easy-to-follow handbook could be a lifesaver if this is the problem you're suffering. The handbook outlines signs and symptoms in more depth while providing scientific research to back Dr. Crook's findings as well as offering dietary, nutritional and medical advice to help people overcome this disease.

You on a Diet: The Owner's Manual for Waist Management

Ref. Roizen, MF, Oz MC. *You on a Diet: The Owner's Manuel for Waist Management*. New York, NY: Free Press, 2009.

Written by the extremely popular Michael F. Roizen, MD, and Mehmet C. Oz, MD. Skyrocketing to fame on the Oprah Show, Dr. Oz is a voice in many households. Popularity aside, this is an incredibly well-written and easy-to-understand book. Through simple text and pictures, You on a Diet explains how the body works, what makes us fat, and what we can do about it. Also included are exercise routines and recipes that reduce fat and inflammation in the body. I really like this book because it helps the not-so-science-inclined person understand how his or her body works -- incredibly important if we are to stay healthy.

Notes

PAGE

1-2 Americans spend more money per person… and following statistics as well as the "Facts." Campbell, TC and Campbell, TM. *The China Study: Startling Implications for Diet, Weight Loss and Long-Term Health*. Dallas, TX: BenBella Books, 006.

9 Research shows the lowest incidence… Robbins, J. The Food Revolution. Berkeley, CA: Conari Press, 2001.

9-10 All "Facts." Robbins J. *The Food Revolution*. Berkeley, CA: Conari Press, 2001.

10 The average IQ of vegetarian children… Robbins, J. *The Food Revolution*. Berkeley, CA: Conari Press, 2001.

11-12 "Facts." Campbell, TC and Campbel,l TM. *The China Study: Startling Implications for Diet, Weight Loss and Long-Term Health*. Dallas, TX: BenBella Books, 2006.

13 "Facts." Robbins, J. The Food Revolution. Berkeley, CA: Conari Press, 2001.

16 Over 1 million Americans will undergo… Robbins, J. *The Food Revolution*. Berkeley, CA: Conari Press, 2001.

17 If we suffer with high blood pressure we are… Robbins, J. *The Food Revolution*. Berkeley, CA: Conari Press, 2001.

17 The truth is that cancer drugs... Robbins, J. *The Food Revolution*. Berkeley, CA: Conari Press, 2001.

18 "Facts." Robbins, J. *The Food Revolution*. Berkeley, CA: Conari Press, 2001.

20 "Facts." Robbins, J. *The Food Revolution*. Berkeley, CA: Conari Press, 2001.

PAGE

22 Scientific evidence also shows that HFCS increases... Weil, A. *Eating Well For Optimum Health*. New York, NY: Alfred A. Knopf, Inc., 2001.

23 "Facts." Robbins, J. The Food Revolution. Berkeley, CA: Conari Press, 2001.

33 Stress is said to account for up to 80 percent... Benson, H. *The Relaxation Response*. New York, NY: HarperTorch, 2000.

34 It is estimated that over 70 percent of people... Rossman, ML. *Guided Imagery for Self-Healing*. Tiburon, CA: H J Kramer, 2000.

40 Research shows that about 40 percent of Americans... Institute of Medicine. *Sleep Disorders and Sleep Deprivation: An Unmet Public Health Problem*. Washington, DC: The National Academies Press; 2006.

51 For example, it is estimated that you would... Robbins, J. *The Food Revolution*. Berkeley, CA: Conari Press, 2001.

Appendix A was adapted from:

Crook, WG. The Yeast Connection Handbook. Jackson, TN: Professional Books, Inc, 2002.

www.ingramcontent.com/pod-product-compliance
Ingram Content Group UK Ltd.
Pitfield, Milton Keynes, MK11 3LW, UK
UKHW020139250726
13967UKWH00002B/742

9 781467 599306